An Integrated View of Health and Well-being

Cross-Cultural Advancements in Positive Psychology

Volume 5

The aim of the *Cross Cultural Advancements in Positive Psychology* book series is to spread a universal and culture-fair perspective on good life promotion. The series will advance a deeper understanding of the cross-cultural differences in well-being conceptualization. A deeper understanding can affect psychological theories, interventions and social policies in various domains, from health to education, from work to leisure. Books in the series will investigate such issues as enhanced mobility of people across nations, ethnic conflicts and the challenges faced by traditional communities due to the pervasive spreading of modernization trends. New instruments and models will be proposed to identify the crucial components of well-being in the process of acculturation. This series will also explore dimensions and components of happiness that are currently overlooked because happiness research is grounded in the Western tradition, and these dimensions do not belong to the Western cultural frame of mind and values.

For further volumes:
http://www.springer.com/series/8420

Antonio Morandi • A.N. Narayanan Nambi
Editors

An Integrated View of Health and Well-being

Bridging Indian and Western Knowledge

Springer

Editors
Antonio Morandi
Ayurvedic Point
Milano, Italy

A.N. Narayanan Nambi
SNA Oushadhasala Pvt. Ltd
Thrissur, Kerala, India

ISSN 2210-5417 ISSN 2210-5425 (electronic)
ISBN 978-94-007-6688-4 ISBN 978-94-007-6689-1 (eBook)
DOI 10.1007/978-94-007-6689-1
Springer Dordrecht Heidelberg New York London

Library of Congress Control Number: 2013939611

Printed on acid-free paper

Springer is part of Springer Science+Business Media (www.springer.com)

Introduction

Antonio Morandi and A.N. Narayanan Nambi

Health, health care, and well-being promotion are pillars of any human social system. However, the social representations of the body, the mind, and their pathologies are strongly influenced by cultural norms and beliefs. The culture of India is a melting pot of diverse philosophical visions translated in practical terms. Historically, Indian tradition comprises nine main philosophical systems, or *Dharshana*, which were formalized between the tenth century BC and the fourth century AD. In spite of their differences, these systems of thought pragmatically coexisted in the foundation and building of Indian culture, sharing a common core that is the realization of the self in the society. The traditional health system of India – Āyurveda – has been elaborated and formalized throughout the centuries as a practical application of the *Dharshana* to the observation of human nature and behavior.

Āyurveda conceptualizes health, disease, and well-being as multidimensional aspects of life, bringing philosophical principles into practice. Its approach to health is basically integrated: in order to attain an optimal adaptation, individuals should preserve a balance at the biological and psychological level, as well at the level of their interaction with environmental demands. This balance is dynamic, and it is based on the interplay between the specific individual biopsychic constitution on the one hand and the ceaseless solicitations derived from the natural and social context on the other hand. The harmonization of individuals' needs and growth tendencies with the environmental requirements fosters health and well-being.

This approach is remarkably close to the conceptualization of well-being proposed by the most recent advancements in psychology, in particular to the eudaemonic

A. Morandi (✉)
Ayurvedic Point, Milano, Italy
e-mail: dr.morandi@ayurvedicpoint.it

A.N. Narayanan Nambi
SNA Oushadhasala Pvt. Ltd, Thrissur, Kerala, India
e-mail: drnambi@hotmail.com

approach developed within positive psychology. Moreover, the basic tenets of Āyurveda are deeply consistent with the latest acquisitions in modern physics, which stresses the substantial interconnectedness among natural phenomena and their substrates. Finally, the growing emphasis of Western medicine on the bio-psycho-social dimensions of health and the increasing claim for an integrated approach to the treatment of chronic and degenerative diseases make the exploration of synergies and complementarities among different healing systems a necessary step. This book shows how the approach to health developed in Āyurveda can be useful and fruitfully integrated in a general, global model of health and well-being encompassing cultural and ideological boundaries. In particular, the conceptualization of health as an optimal and mindful interaction between individuals and their environment will be discussed as the core of a new paradigm of healthy life and behavior.

The book is articulated into four parts. The reader will be guided in a conceptual journey that, moving from the Western perspective, will cross the immense land of Indian knowledge, reaching a crossroad where an integration of the two approaches will be proposed. The classical Ayurvedic texts cited and referred to in the chapters of the second part comprise three main works: *Ćaraka Saṃhitā*, *Suśruta Saṃhitā*, and *Aṣṭāṅga Hṛdaya*. These treatises, which were composed between the seventh century BC and the sixth century AD, are considered the pillars of Āyurveda teachings and practice.

Part I: Health and Well-Being in the Western Tradition

Corey L. M. Keyes and Kate Cartwright open the book with "Well-Being in the West: Hygieia Before and After the Demographic Transition" (Chap. 1), an overview of the historical and social factors that led to the current Western conceptualization of health and disease. The Western culture inherited from ancient Greeks a dual view of health – as the absence of illness (the pathogenic view, Panacea) and as a positive event referred to as well-being (the salutogenic view, Hygieia). The modifications in fertility-mortality ratios that occurred throughout time, and the associated economic changes, generated a swinging cycle of pathogenic and salutogenic views of health. The increased citizens' expectations related to a longer life expectancy favor a growing attention to the identification of the causes of disease. At the same time, the phenomenon of population aging, with its burden of chronic and age-related problems, orients researchers' interest and governments' investments toward prevention practices and quality of life improvement. Western society is in fact facing the inappropriateness of the Panacea, disease-focused approach. Moreover, the steadily increasing costs of health care make the switch to the salutogenic approach mandatory. These considerations point to a broader conceptualization of health, encompassing social and economic factors, as well as psychological dimensions and their interplay with physical health.

Nicoletta Sonino and Giovanni A. Fava in "The Psychosomatic View" (Chap. 2) describe one of the most rigorous approaches developed in the West to promote the salutogenic view of health. Psychosomatic medicine takes into account the multifactorial determinants of health, with the aim to integrate psychological dimension in the clinical practice. It considers the patient from a bio-psycho-social point of view, emphasizing the importance of lifestyle and psychological balance for a healthy living. Noteworthy, its conceptual framework represents an important point of convergence between the Western and the Eastern medical approaches.

Part II: Health and Well-Being in Indian Traditions

Kiran Kumar K. Salagame in "The Perspectives on Reality in Indian Traditions and Their Implications for Health and Well-Being" (Chap. 3) analyzes the differences between the Western and Indian perspectives of reality and their influence on the vision of health and disease in the two cultures. He also points to the changes undergoing in the Western reductionistic view that is moving from a biomedical disease-centered model toward a different conceptualization of health and well-being. In this context the Indian system of knowledge and representation of reality is proposed as a paradigm endorsing a holistic view of human nature and thus supporting the adoption of intervention strategies aimed at pursuing prevention and optimal health and well-being, rather than disease treatment. Among the health-related knowledge systems of India, Āyurveda, the ancient traditional medicine, is the most codified and representative, and its model of health is consistent with the paradigm described by K.K.K. Salagame.

Ram Manohar in "Concept of Health in Āyurveda" (Chap. 4) discusses the Ayurvedic vision of health as the integration of body, mind, and spirit, whose interplay defines the individual's interaction with the environment and its changes. Processes such as psycho-spiritual growth and awareness are fundamental to establish individual and social health and well-being.

The conceptualization of health and disease that characterizes Āyurveda is further discussed by A.N. Narayanan Nambi in "Determinants of Health and Well-Being in Āyurveda" (Chap. 5). This chapter analyzes the "bodies" identified by Āyurveda – gross, mental, and subtle – and their interrelationships, from which the experience of life, health, and well-being derive. The chapter emphasizes the inherent interconnectedness between macrocosm and microcosm, humans and environment, and the role of individual awareness and behavior in the fine-tuned regulation of this interaction. In this view, mental and behavioral adequacy represents the inner determinants of health and well-being.

The phenomenon of rituals in Indian culture and their relationship with health is analyzed by P.R. Krishna Kumar in "The Role of Social Rituals in Well-Being" (Chap. 6). Community rituals contribute to social well-being as behaviors that carry information useful to maintain the correct relationship of each individual with the environment and with other members of the community. The order principle underlying these relations in their ideal structure is the core of the concept of *dharma*. Warning is also made to the risk of fixation and rigidity of rituals, which makes them not only ineffective but also detrimental to the regulation of human actions and transactions.

A further analysis of health-related traditional values and customs is conducted by Unnikrishnan Payyappallimana in "Health and Well-Being in Indian Local Health Traditions" (Chap. 7). He analyzes the amazing diversity and plurality of knowledge systems and traditions originated from the likewise mottled set of ecosystems and human activities that characterize the Indian subcontinent, with specific attention to health systems. The coexistence and deep interplay of oral and codified knowledge have generated deeply rooted and sophisticated cultural practices, in particular with regard to health. Attention is paid to the links and to the shared elements of and codified health systems across diverse communities in Southern India.

Part III: Bridging the Worlds

Western scientific research conducted in the last few decades brought about new insights and models in the conceptualization of living systems and their functioning. The attempt to integrate in the scientific domain psychological, social, and spiritual dimensions is supported by concepts such as indetermination and interconnectedness, which are not necessarily legitimated by sensory perception.

Rama Jayasundar in "Quantum Logic in Āyurveda" (Chap. 8) reviews the parallels existing between the model of reality proposed by quantum physics and the Vedic knowledge and highlights the potential of Āyurveda to integrate their common elements in a shared view. The basic common element of the two models is the ontological unity and interconnectedness of everything in the universe. The individual is an indivisible network of relationships continuously promoting information exchange within and without the body at different levels, including mind and consciousness, which play a central role in maintaining the balance of the system. The balance or the unbalance of these relationships defines the state or level of health. The important contribution of the chapter is represented by the suggestion that through Āyurveda it is possible to put into practice the common principles underlying both quantum physics and Vedic logic.

The importance of individual agency and responsibility in health management is specifically stressed by Antonella Delle Fave in "The Psychological Roots of Health Promotion" (Chap. 9). The chapter examines the psychological dimensions of health as identified within the framework of the Western bio-psycho-social model, drawing parallels and highlighting connections with the Āyurveda's model of health, which similarly stresses the primacy of psychological variables on physical ones in health management. While acknowledging cultural differences, a substantial convergence is shown between the bio-psycho-social model and Āyurveda, with particular regard to the pivotal role of individuals as main agents and determinants of their own health.

Nevertheless, a further integration of the two systems would be welcome, especially considering the potential contribution of Āyurveda in promoting an active and aware prevention based on the articulated conceptual framework of interconnectedness. In order to pursue this integration, deeper levels of analysis are needed with the aim of identifying the fundamental principles and logic shared by the two systems. However, from the Western perspective, little is still understood of the reality framework described in Āyurveda. Its inclusive logic is not easily understandable according to Western scientific principles. To fill this gap and to infer a possible, integrated definition of health, Antonio Morandi and Antonella Delle Fave propose an original approach in their chapter "The Emergence of Health in Complex Adaptive Systems: A Common Ground for Āyurveda and Western Science" (Chap. 10). After an overview of the complex system logical framework, they discuss the inclusive logic underpinning Āyurveda and its model of reality, exemplified through a thorough description of the living beings' components. These authors suggest the convergence of the Western and Indian perspectives in the view of individuals as complex adaptive systems, and of health as a phenomenon emerging from their dynamic bio-psycho-social balance. The theoretical and practical implications of this approach pave the way to a unified and integrated vision of health, overcoming the boundaries between disciplines and cultures.

Contents

Part I
Health and Well-Being in the Western Tradition

Chapter 1
Well-Being in the West: Hygieia Before and After the Demographic Transition

Corey L.M. Keyes and Kate Cartwright

1.1 Introduction

The Greek physicians and philosophers have been the inspiration for much of the thinking and approaches to health and illness in the modern world. Hart's (1965) classic article ascribes the origin myth of modern medicine to the cult of Asclepius, a deity in ancient Greece who is known as the father of medicine. As the story goes, Asclepius gave birth to several daughters, two of whom represented the distinct but complementary branches of medicine. The daughter named *Panacea* represented the branch of medicine that focused on the remediation of illness, while the other daughter named *Hygieia* represented the branch of medicine devoted to the promotion of good health. To this day, the staff of Asclepius represents the symbol of medicine, the snake that winds itself around the staff represents good health (i.e., Hygieia, because the snake regularly sheds its skin in the process of reestablishing its health), and the Hippocratic oath taken by all new medical doctors swears allegiance to Asclepius and to both branches of medicine—panacea and hygieia (see Hart 1965).

In short, we in the West inherited a view of health from the ancient Greeks as being more than the absence of illness. However, until very recently, health as something positive, or what we will refer to as "well-being," has not been central to any discussion of medical practice or to population health. In practice, most Western approaches to health have focused almost exclusively on understanding pathogenesis, or the origin and cause of illness or disease. The dominant view of health in the West is that health is the absence of disease and illness. This view of health has not gone unchallenged, but this challenge began only recently in the twentieth century as a result of the rise of research on well-being that reflected the need to recover the hygienic perspective rooted in the myth of Asclepius that health is the presence of positive qualities and capacities.

C.L.M. Keyes (✉) • K. Cartwright
Department of Sociology, Emory University, Atlanta, GA, USA
e-mail: ckeyes@emory.edu

A. Morandi and A.N. Narayanan Nambi (eds.), *An Integrated View of Health and Well-being*, Cross-Cultural Advancements in Positive Psychology 5, DOI 10.1007/978-94-007-6689-1_1,

The scientific study of well-being arose during the last third of the twentieth century in the USA and has blossomed since then and brought increased attention for the need to engage in promotion of good health in the population. In this chapter, we will argue that the fall of hygieia occurs during the initial stage of the demographic transition in nations, when economic development hastens and then sets off a sequence of changes called the demographic transition (Omran 1971) that results in an increased population and life expectancy. The changes begin with the reduction of deaths in the population that occurs while fertility rates remain high for a prolonged period. During this period, the population of a nation increases, often dramatically. In the wake of the population growth, changes occur in education and contraception that usher in a reduction in rates of fertility in the population.

During this time when mortality declines and, later, fertility declines, the causes of disease and death are also transformed from acute and infectious conditions to chronic and preventable conditions. The result is increased pressure on the economic development of a nation due to a larger population, an aging population that is also living longer but often with chronic conditions that, though preventable, are now managed through expensive medical systems which were originally designed to deal not with chronic illness but with acute conditions (further discussion of these topics can be found in Chaps. 9 and 10 of this volume). Early in the stage of the transition, medicalization, we argue, shifts away from the "art" of well-being or positive health (i.e., away from Hygieia) and moves toward a strict scientific focus on pathogenesis and illness (i.e., the rise of panacea). As the later stage of this transition, the changes in life expectancy, causes of illness and death, and the aging of the population place pressure on the economic system of a country that requires, we argue, a return in focus on hygienic or well-being promoting activities that prevent chronic conditions and physical and mental illness.

1.2 The Rise of Panacea and Demise of Hygieia

1.2.1 Rapid Industrialization and Urbanization of Europe and the USA

Although the majority of disease reduction in the modern Western world is attributable to advancements relating to *hygieia* (i.e., prevention), principles and practices of *panacea* dominate contemporary Western medicine. This section of the chapter addresses the question of what led to the rise of panacea in Western medicine and what implications does this emphasis have on the profession of medicine and its outcomes. The eighteenth and nineteenth centuries were periods of revolution in the Western world: political, scientific, industrial, communication, transportation, and agricultural. Along with the rapid industrialization and urbanization of Europe came waves of concentrated illness including cholera, smallpox, and tuberculosis. Societies were faced with high mortality rates, higher for the urban poor, and these illnesses and mortality rates yielded the development of public health and the institutionalization of modern medicine (Porter 2002; Starr 1982; Weitz 2010).

Due to advancements in public health and structural changes, such as sewer systems, water treatment systems and advancements in general hygiene, deaths from infectious diseases decreased rapidly by the end of the nineteenth century. This led to important changes in society. Primarily, families had fewer children, as the probability that the children would live to adulthood was much greater and the vocational shift from agriculture to industry decreased the need for large families. Due to smaller family sizes, more resources were available to each member. More resources and a decrease in infectious diseases led to greater life expectancy.

Progress in modern medicine led to the rationalization and bureaucratization that continues to frame Western medicine today. Although evidence suggests that principles of hygieia were primarily responsible for the reduction of these illnesses (McKinlay and McKinlay 1977), the emergent zeitgeist called for treatments and cures, leading to the rise of panacea as the dominant focus of Western medicine. While there is more balance in the hygieia/panacea continuum in some nations, the contemporary focus of Western medicine continues to be on panacea.

1.2.2 Rationalization and Bureaucratization of Medicine

The institutionalization of medicine in the Western world accompanied the rationalization and bureaucratization of medicine. Before institutionalization, medicine was practiced in more individualized ways and in more private of spaces, like patients' homes. By the mid-nineteenth century, the differentiation of medical spaces was firmly established. Instead of a patient's home being the primary site of medical practice, there were a number of formally legitimated spaces for medicine: the doctor's office, medical universities, hospitals, morgues, and laboratories (Rothman et al. 1995).

As medicine advanced and knowledge became more widely agreed upon and widespread, what constituted good medicine became standardized. The nineteenth century ushered in the rationalization of many societal institutions. Primarily, rationalization of medicine worked to organize principles and practices into a standardized system and rationale based on scientifically derived guidelines. Bureaucratization accompanied the continuing development of division of labor that gave different workers specialized roles in a hierarchy intended to streamline a process and keep a system accountable and reliable. Rationalization and bureaucratization in society became prevalent as means to promote equality, in the spirit of developing democracy and efficiency in societies that valued progress (Weber 1947). They also resulted in the commodification of many services that had previously never been considered a commodity. This shift affected Western medicine greatly.

Prior to the rationalization and bureaucratization of medicine, doctors largely worked independently, and their work was viewed as a service. However, rationalization and bureaucratization led to society viewing medicine as a potential business and health as a commodity to be sold (Starr 1982). This further led to an emphasis on panacea, as peddling a treatment or a cure fit into the paradigm of supply and demand much better than the more abstract concepts of prevention, regardless of the fact that prevention offered the most efficient and reliable practices and outcomes. A treatment or a cure offers a tangible product for which individuals have a clear demand. In order to build a market for this product, the places where medicine was practiced changed and the process of medicine shifted. An emphasis on panacea and the rationalization and bureaucratization of medicine led to the development of medicalized spaces, such as hospitals and doctors' offices, and the formalization of the diagnostic process. Hospitals shifted from being primarily institutions for the poor to centers of scientific advancement in medicine (Porter 2002). Along with the development of hospitals came the rise of the nursing profession. The focus on treatment was reliant on the ability to correctly diagnose an ailment, which created a demand for more skilled diagnosticians and a more reliable diagnostic process.

The development of diagnostic medicine shifted Western medicine from a patient-centered practice to a doctor-centered one. Instead of valuing and prioritizing information provided by patients, doctors focused on their own medical examination and prioritized information gleaned from this practice to determine the patient's condition (Numbers 2001). The emphasis on diagnosis made disease and not the patient the subject of medical intervention. The practice of diagnosis combined with a business model of medicine created the dynamic in which the question of what is wrong with the patient became more important than why is something wrong. The "what" question leads to a culture of treatment and cures, which promotes not only the diagnostic field of medicine but also the business of pharmaceuticals.

This helps explain why diagnosis and the scientific method value cures over prevention. As the work of a doctor stems from an ability to diagnose and treat illness, the highest levels of status and prestige are given to doctors who can cure or treat the most difficult and rare conditions, as opposed to emphasizing lifestyles that would prevent common ailments. This is particularly true for the American medical culture. The payment structure of many Western nations reaffirms these priorities, as it compensates doctors and medical professionals for particular diagnoses and treatments at a much greater rate than prevention. The development of diagnostic medicine led not only to a more standardized practice of medicine but also to a standardized process of medical training, leading to a more formal professionalization of the field.

1.2.3 The Professionalization of Medicine

The rise and development of the medical profession is central to the current focus of treatment and cures dominating contemporary Western medicine. Medical education developed in the eighteenth century, which led to the establishment of medical schools throughout the Western world. Formal education helped to legitimize the field of medicine and practitioners such as physicians, surgeons, and pharmacists became licensed. Along with professionalization of the field came prestige. Society began to revere medical professionals instead of treating them with suspicion (Numbers 2001). The job of healing shifted from being widely spread among different entities to being carefully controlled. While these professions rose in prestige, other healing professions, such as religious healers, herbalists, and mid-wifes, became delegitimized, and formal steps were put in place to prevent these non-authorized healers from practicing medicine. Western nations passed acts that regulated the licensure of medical professionals, such as the 1858 British Medical Act (Starr 1982). As a result of the rationalization of medicine, medical associations were formed in the nineteenth century that authorized and monitored medical professionals.

The legitimation of the medical field and the professionalization of medicine highlighted the inequality of status and knowledge between doctor and patient, which continues to influence contemporary dynamics. With the rising authority of medicine, previously "normal" conditions, such as birth, many life events (including menopause), and death become medicalized. Instead of being considered as expected events for which most people's bodies are prepared and which primarily could take place in one's home, these conditions came to require hospital stays and bureaucratic procedures that made life more convenient for doctors as opposed to being medically necessary. Childbirth practices in the United States are a good example of a common condition that has become over-medicalized. The United States has the highest rate of caesarean section births, reaching 32.3 % in 2008 (Martin et al. 2010). While the increase in this rate is in part related to an increase in higher risk births (including births to older women, women with obesity and diabetes issues, and an increase in multiples due to fertility treatments), other nonclinical factors including maternal choice, physician scheduling, and medico-legal pressures are large contributing forces behind this trend (Martin et al. 2010). This is an expected result of a rationalized and highly bureaucratic society that transforms a process, which was intended to make a procedure safer, more efficient, and more egalitarian, into a procedure for procedure's sake. While this practice may be more efficient and predictable, especially for doctors on tight schedules, statistics show that it is not safer for mother or child and it is not being practiced in an egalitarian manner. Mothers have a greater risk of post-pregnancy complications after a caesarean section; infants are more frequently born preterm, thus being exposed to a greater risk for a variety of short-term and long-term health challenges. Experts are so concerned about this practice in the United States that a number of investigations have been conducted and goals for decreasing the caesarean rate have been set. Caesarean section births have risen in all Western nations in the past 30 years, but while some nations have higher rates than the United States (also Italy and Australia), many other Western nations with more collective health-care systems and systems focused more directly on outcomes have much lower rates (the United Kingdom, Norway, and Sweden). The privatization of medicine in the United States seems to have directly contributed to an increase in the over-medicalization of the practice of childbirth.

Another contributor to the rise in medicalization of conditions is Western medicine's focus on specialists (Starr 1982). Along with the professionalization and progress of medical fields came a division of labor that separated general practitioners from specialists. On average, specialists are regarded with higher prestige and are compensated at greater rates, even though many of them treat conditions that afflict a small percentage of the population. Of course, it is a testament to the amazing capabilities of modern medicine that specialists are able to perform highly complex interventions such as brain surgery, organ transplants, and treatment of difficult forms of cancer. However, the focus on specializations in Western medicine raises the prestige of medical doctors who can perform the most complicated and dangerous procedures and diminishes the role of the general practitioner who has the ability to affect the most people and prevent the most disease. This is both a product of and a reification of Western medicine's focus on panacea as opposed to hygieia.

1.2.4 The Rise and Role of Pharmaceuticals

If the nineteenth century established the superiority and authority of the doctor, the twentieth century marked the legitimization of the pharmaceutical industry. While the pharmaceutical profession had been growing, the potential for pharmaceuticals to dominate the market was not fully realized until the twentieth century. Of course, panaceas were peddled throughout the development of Western medicine, but only after the epidemiological transition from infectious disease to chronic disease pharmaceuticals became a part of everyday life (Weitz 2010). As infectious diseases waned, chronic pathologies such as hypertension, diabetes, and heart disease grew. These diseases could not be cured (although they could be prevented with lifestyle changes), but through the development of drugs, they could be managed. The pharmaceutical industry experienced the same rationalization and bureaucratization as the rest of Western medicine, and the majority of national drug administrations came into existence in the early twentieth century.

The US Food and Drug Administration (FDA) was founded in 1906, and this led to many positive outcomes in regard to quality regulation of drugs and accountability of the pharmaceutical industry. The development of the pharmaceutical industry also differentiated types of drugs (prescription, generic, vitamins, food supplements, homeopathic medicines) and created a market for advertising. To some degree, marketing influences all of Western medicine (as also highlighted in Chap. 3 of this volume). This is particularly true of the United States, where direct-to-patient consumer advertising of pharmaceuticals is allowed, but also where the most powerful marketing industries are settled. This affects the doctor-patient relationship, as the patient is more likely to come in requesting information and perhaps prescriptions for certain drugs.

1.2.5 The Social Meaning of Illness

In addition to scientific advances in medicine, social and cultural values play an important role in the principles and practice of Western medicine. The range of theories and practices employed by physicians is scientifically based and motivated, but it is embedded within evolving cultures and values. In order to best understand Western medicine, it is important to understand the social construction of disease in Western societies. In this context, the medical model of illness stems from the scientific method, where disease is determined by conditions that deviate from the norms of health and is caused by unique biological forces. Definitions and classifications of disease and conditions come from and are treated through an unbiased scientific process (Weitz 2010). Throughout the history of Western medicine, however, values, politics, and other social forces have influenced conceptions of the nature of disease, of health, and of medicine.

The sociological perspective incorporates those social forces into the discussion of what medicine is, acknowledging that illness is socially constructed and that it exists because society has made it so. In addition to our discussion of childbirth and pharmaceutically led disease mongering, another good example of this is the journey of homosexuality. In the nineteenth century, homosexuality was medicalized as well as pathologized as a mental illness. This classification was fraught with value judgments and was not based on evidence from an "unbiased scientific process". It was given even more authority when it was included in the Diagnostic and Statistical Manual (DSM) of mental disorders in 1952. However, as values and culture shifted, homosexuality experienced a de-medicalization and de-pathologization, and it was removed from the DSM in 1974. The case of homosexuality shows that diagnosis is not an objective, neutral, scientific process, but in fact is influenced by a variety of social forces. Social forces are also evident in the disparities of diagnoses. Frequently patients with the same symptoms receive different diagnoses and differential treatment based not on comorbidities or scientific risk factors but on factors such as race, gender, and class. Nations with nationalized health care run lower risks of differential treatment based on financial resources, although these systems are not immune to class bias in treatment either. For example, health-care providers are products of their particular social situations, and these situations bias the way in which doctors perform medicine. This makes the focus on panacea in Western medicine even more problematic, because biases and social forces lead to a disparity in treatment for different social groups and the panaceas produced are unequally available. Means of mediating these biases include the adoption of nationalized health-care systems, diagnostic audits of doctors, and studies of health disparities in a society. Another way to prevent disparity in treatment of disease is to shift from a focus on panacea to hygieia and prevent the conditions that need treatment in the first place.

1.3 Return of Hygieia and Well-Being in the West

The rise of panacea corresponds to a focus on the *quantity* of life, because most research on pathogenesis represent an attempt to reduce the leading, and more proximal, causes of premature death. That is, extended life expectancy is among the leading goals during the rise of panacea. However, the return of Hygieia, which includes a return to well-being, represents a shift toward the goal to increase the *quality* of life.

The quality of an individual's life can be assessed externally and objectively or internally and subjectively. From an objective standpoint, other people measure and judge another's life according to criteria such as wealth or income, educational attainment, occupational prestige, and health status or longevity. Nations, communities, or individuals who are wealthier, have more education, and live longer are considered to have higher quality of life or personal well-being. The subjective standpoint emerged during the 1950s as an important alternative to the objective approach to measuring individual's well-being. Subjectively, individuals evaluate their own lives after reviewing, summing, and weighing their substance. In short, subjective well-being is an evaluation or declaration that individuals make about the quality of their lives (Diener et al. 1999; Keyes et al. 2002).

Well-being has been a paramount concern of thinkers since ancient times, as witnessed in much of Greek philosophical writings on the nature and pursuit of happiness or the good life. Subjective well-being became a topic of scientific inquiry during the 1950s when interest in fostering a better life was facilitated by the Zeitgeist following World War II. The world's recovery from the manifold devastation—physical, psychological, social, and moral—of the war encouraged commitment to social welfare, greater attention to the diversity of people and viewpoints, and greater appreciation of the individual. This atmosphere manifested itself in philosophical (e.g., phenomenology and existentialism), sociological (e.g., symbolic interactionism), and psychological (e.g., cognitive psychology and later the focus on emotions) movements that focused on the centrality of the individual's perceptions and viewpoints and the importance of personal meaning and concerns about life.

Subjective well-being therefore emerged as a scientific field in the late 1950s, when social scientists developed indicators of quality of life to monitor social change and to improve social policy (Land 1975) as well as pursue a more humanistic scientific agenda. Humanistic writings emphasized several concerns and constructs that buttressed the study of subjective well-being. In reaction to the negative portrayal of human nature and potential in orthodox psychoanalysis, humanistic scholars catalogued the individual's capacity for successful adjustment through the development of positive characteristics such as maturity, ego-strength, generativity, and virtues (see e.g., Erik Erikson's writings) (Erikson 1950, 1959). In reaction to the hegemony of behaviorism's focus on only observable behavior as data, humanistic writers lauded introspection and subjective appraisal as meaningful data. Humanistic social scientists sought to understand whole lives by investigating how individuals felt about their own lives. This strand of humanism was exemplified in the methods of many personality psychologists, notably Gordon Allport (cited in Severin 1965), who declared that

> It is not enough to know how man reacts: we must know how he feels, how he sees his world, … why he lives, what he fears, for what he would be willing to die. Such questions of *existence* must be put to man directly. (p. 42)

In other words, introspection and self-reports on one' own feelings and outlook were once again important and legitimate sources of scientific data.

During this same historical period, the US Congress passed the "Mental Health Act" that earmarked future funds for the creation of a "National Institute of Mental Health" (NIMH), which was slated to come into being in 1949. The joint commission on mental health and illness, which served as the advisory board for the creation of the future NIMH, contained the intellectual seeds of the two dominant streams of research on subjective well-being today. This commission, chaired and dominated by psychiatrists, requested several reports ranging from the state of mental health services to epidemiology of mental health and illness. Though clearly in the minority, several Ph.D.s, including M. Brewster Smith (1959), were responsible for publishing two separate reports on mental health, both of which reported on the status of theory and research on subjective well-being.

The first publication was Marie Jahoda's (1958) seminal volume on positive mental health. This volume reviewed the personality and clinical psychology literatures regarding dimensions of psychological well-being (e.g., purpose in life, personal growth, and self-acceptance) that reflected aspects of eudaimonic stream of subjective well-being. The second volume, in terms of its publication, was Gurin et al. (1960) book on the state of American's mental health. It featured the hedonic stream of subjective well-being with its focus on individuals' assessments of their satisfaction and happiness with life, overall and in specific domains of life (e.g., work and family).

Notwithstanding this focus on subjective well-being and not only mental illness, the Mental Health Act of 1946 gave way in title only to the National Institute of Mental *Health*. In practice and programs, the NIMH remains committed to the promotion of America's mental health through the study of the etiology and treatment of mental *illness*. Although subjective well-being did not become part of this nation's mental health agenda, the impetus to launch the NIMH may have responsible for planting the seeds of the study of subjective well-being as it appears today in the traditions of eudaimonic and hedonic well-being (Ryff 1989; Ryff and Keyes 1995; Keyes et al. 2002).

Since Jahoda's (1958) and Gurin et al.'s (1960) seminal work, social science scholars (psychologists, sociologists, and economists) have spent the past 40 years moving forward the nascent agenda of mental health via the study of subjective well-being. In the 1980s, two seminal journal articles brought the study of subjective well-being and its two traditions into the mainstream of social psychological inquiry. The first was Ed Diener's (1984) review article of the state of the first generation of research and theory on subjective well-being, which had focused squarely on hedonic dimensions, such as happiness, life satisfaction, or affect balance. The second was Carol Ryff's (1989) article that operationalized the theory of psychological well-being outlined in Jahoda's (1958) volume and argued that happiness is not merely hedonic but also includes eudaimonic elements. These influential and highly cited articles revitalized the traditions of subjective well-being research that form the basis for much the today's research on subjective well-being.

Until the late 1980s, research on subjective well-being was synonymous with hedonic well-being (Kahneman et al. 1999). Despite this prejudice to equate subjective well-being with hedonic happiness (Ryff 1989), new research clearly shows that subjective well-being is a multifactorial, multidimensional concept. One result of the nearly 50 years of research on this important concept is that researchers have proliferated, by my count (Keyes 2005a), at least 13 dimensions of subjective well-being in the United States. Moreover, research has confirmed the meta-theoretical hypothesis of hedonic and eudaimonic traditions of thought and functioning that inform the study of subjective well-being (Keyes et al. 2002; King and Napa 1998; Ryan and Deci 2001; Ryff 1989; Waterman 1990, 1993).

Hedonic, or emotional, well-being is a specific dimension of subjective well-being that consists of perceptions of avowed interest in life, happiness and satisfaction with life, and the balance of positive to negative affect (Bradburn 1969; Bryant and Veroff 1982; Cantril 1965; Diener et al. 1985; Lucas et al. 1996; Shmotkin 1998). In contrast, eudaimonic well-being, sometimes referred to as positive functioning, consists of individual's evaluation of their psychological well-being (Ryff 1989; Ryff and Keyes 1995).

A variety of concepts from personality, developmental, and clinical psychology have been synthesized as criteria of mental health (Jahoda 1958) and psychological well-being (Ryff 1989). Elements of psychological well-being are descended from the Aristotle's position on happiness as eudaimonia, which states that the highest of all goods achievable deliberately by humans is the development of a good life, which mirrors concepts such as self-actualization (Maslow 1968), full functioning (Rogers 1961), individuation (Jung 1933), maturity (Allport 1961), and successful adult development that results in the realization of virtues (Erikson 1959). Ryff (1989) integrated these writing into psychometrically sound measures reflecting a multidimensional model of psychological well-being. Each of the six dimensions of psychological well-being indicates the challenges that individuals encounter as they strive to function fully and realize their unique talents (see Keyes and Ryff 1999; Ryff 1989; Ryff and Keyes 1995). The six dimensions encompass a breadth of well-being: positive evaluation of oneself and one's past life, a sense of continued growth and development as a person, the belief that one's life is purposeful and meaningful, the possession of quality relations with others, the capacity to manage effectively one's life and surrounding world, and a sense of self-determination (Ryff and Keyes 1995).

Within the eudaimonic tradition, there was scant recognition of the social dimensions of an individual's functioning in life. The quality of individuals' relationships to, and functioning in, society and social groups remains understudied aspects of individuals' health. This is largely the reason why the first author of this chapter initiated a study of social well-being (Keyes 1998), defined as individuals' perceptions of the quality of their relationships with other people, their neighborhoods, and their communities. As predicted theoretically, social well-being is multidimensional, and Americans view the quality of their functioning in life based on whether they see social life as meaningful and understandable (social coherence), see society as possessing potential for growth (social actualization), feel they belong to and are accepted by their communities (social integration), feel they accept other people (social acceptance), and see themselves as having something worthwhile to contribute to society (social contribution). In short, eudaimonia consists of both private and public facets of positive functioning. Whereas psychological well-being is conceptualized as a primarily private phenomenon that is focused on the challenges encountered by adults in their private lives, social well-being represents primarily public phenomenon, focused on the social tasks encountered by adults in their social structures and communities.

1.3.1 Hygieia Enters the Debate About Mental Health and Illness

Mental illness has always been seen as problematic but not as public health issue until 1996, when the World Health Organization published the results of the first Global Burden of Disease study (Murray and Lopez 1996). This study estimated the total contribution of 107 acute and chronic medical conditions and illnesses by including disability in the equation to calculate disability-adjusted life years (DALYs). The DALY reflects the total number of years in a population that were either lived with disability or abbreviated prematurely due to specific physical or mental conditions. Depression was the fourth leading cause of disease burden, accounting for 3.7 % of DALYs in 1990, 4.4 % in 2000, and projected to be 15 % of DALYs by 2020 (Ustun 1999; Ustun et al. 2004). As such, the debate is over as whether mental illness is a serious public health issue—it is.

The biggest issue facing governments is what can and should be done to reduce the number of cases of mental illness and those suffering from it. Most governments choose the de facto approach of providing treatment to more individuals (Chisholm et al. 2004). All evidence points to the fact that the de facto approach is not reducing the prevalence, burden, or early age of onset for mental disorders (Kessler et al. 2005; Insel and Scolnick 2006). A viable alternative is mental health promotion, which seeks to elevate levels of positive mental health and protect against its loss (Davis 2002; Jané-Llopis et al. 2005; Keyes 2007; Secker 1998). Whereas treatment targets those with mental illness, and risk reduction prevention targets those vulnerable to mental illness, mental health promotion targets those with good mental health and those with less than optimal mental health—i.e., all members of a population.

The World Health Organization (WHO 2004) recently highlighted the need to promote positive mental health when it defined mental health positively as " … *a state of well–being in which the individual realizes his or her own abilities, can cope with the normal stresses of life, can work productively and fruitfully, and is able to make a contribution to his or her community*" (p. 12). This is good news, because it means the WHO has caught up with science, where positive mental health has been operationalized under the rubric of subjective well-being, or individuals' evaluations of the quality of their lives.

Table 1.1 Tripartite structure and specific dimensions reflecting positive mental health

Hedonia (i.e., emotional well-being)
Positive affect: cheerful, interested in life, in good spirits, happy, calm and peaceful, full of life
Avowed (or cognitive) affect: life satisfaction or satisfaction with domains of life
Positive psychological functioning (i.e., psychological well-being)
Self-acceptance: holds positive attitudes toward self, acknowledges, likes most parts of self, personality
Personal growth: seeks challenge, has insight into own potential, feels a sense of continued development
Purpose in life: finds own life has a direction and meaning
Environmental mastery: exercises ability to select, manage, and mold personal environs to suit needs
Autonomy: is guided by own, socially accepted, internal standards and values
Positive relations with others: has, or can form, warm, trusting personal relationships
Positive social functioning (i.e., social well-being)
Social acceptance: holds positive attitudes toward, acknowledges, and is accepting of human differences
Social growth (actualization): believes people, groups, and society have potential to grow
Social contribution: sees own daily activities a useful to and valued by society and others
Social coherence: interest in society and social life, and finds them meaningful and somewhat intelligible
Social integration: A sense of belonging to, and comfort and support from, a community

When subjective well-being is measured comprehensively, the tripartite model consisting of emotional, psychological, and social well-being is supported in studies involving US adults (Gallagher et al. 2009), college students (Robitschek and Keyes 2009), and adolescents (Keyes 2006). Table 1.1 therefore includes a description of each dimension of emotional, psychological, and social well-being and is organized theoretically according to the categorization of well-being as either hedonic (representing how good individuals feel about their lives) or eudaimonic (how well individuals perceive themselves functioning psychologically and socially in life).

The 14 signs of well-being in Table 1.1 represent the questions in the Mental Health Continuum "Short Form" (MHC-SF). The MHC-SF was created to address the problem of the diagnostic threshold and to create a version more efficiently administered in epidemiological surveillance. The MHC-SF derives from the long form (MHC-LF) used in the Midlife in the United States (MIDUS) study (Keyes 2002, 2005b). While the MHC-LF consisted of 40 items, the MHC-SF consists of 14 of the most prototypical items representing the construct definition for each facet of well-being. Three items (happy, interested in life, and satisfied) indicate emotional well-being, six items measure the six dimensions of psychological well-being, and five items represent the five dimensions of social well-being. The response option for the short form was changed to measure the frequency (from "never" to "every day") with which respondents experienced each sign of mental health during the past month, which provides a clear standard for the assessment and a categorization of levels of mental health that is similar to the survey assessment of mental major depressive episode according to DSM criteria.

The merger of feeling good about a life in which individuals are functioning well, I have argued (Keyes 2002), constitutes the presence of good mental health. In the same way that depression requires symptoms of *an*hedonia, mental health consists of symptoms of hedonia. But feeling good only, in the same way as feeling sad or losing interest in life, is not sufficient for the diagnosis of a clinical state. Rather, and in the same way that major depression consists of symptoms of *mal*functioning, mental health must also consist of symptoms of positive functioning. In turn, the mental health continuum (Keyes 2002) consists of three diagnostic categories, or levels, of positive mental health: flourishing, moderate, and languishing mental health. Individuals with *flourishing* mental health report feeling at least one measure of hedonic well-being plus six or more of the measures of positive functioning almost every day or every day during the past month. Individuals with *languishing* mental health report feeling at least one measure of hedonic well-being with six or more measures of positive functioning never or maybe once or twice during the past month. Languishing is the absence of mental health—a state of being mentally *un*healthy—which is tantamount to being stuck and stagnant, or feeling empty or that life lacks interest and engagement. Individuals who are neither flourishing nor languishing are diagnosed with *moderate* mental health.

1.3.2 The Two Continua Model: Hygieia and Panacea Are Both Important

The importance of measuring mental health in the same way as mental illness cannot be overstated, because it allows us to finally adequately test the hypothesis that mental health and illness belong to two separate continua. Indeed, mental health promotion and protection is premised on the two continua model, because good mental health is presumed to belong to a separate continuum from mental illness (Health and Welfare Canada 1988). Yet, the studies that did exist on the subject only measured mental health emotionally in terms of life satisfaction or happiness (Greenspoon and Saklofske 2001; Headey et al. 1993; Huppert and Whittington 2003; Masse et al. 1998; Suldo and Shaffer 2008; Veit and Ware 1983). Numerous studies in mainstream psychology of emotion have shown that positive and negative emotions belong to separate continua (e.g., Bradburn 1969; Watson and Clark 1997), but as mentioned earlier, emotional disturbance or emotional vitality does not, in themselves, constitute states of mental illness or mental health.

Findings based MHC-LF in the MIDUS study (Keyes 2005b) support the two continua model: One continuum indicates the presence and absence of positive mental health, and the other indicates the presence and absence of mental illness symptoms. For example, though the latent factors of mental illness and mental health correlated ($r=-.53$), only 28.1 % of their variance is shared in the MIDUS data (Keyes 2005a). The two continua model has been replicated in a nationally representative sample of US adolescents (ages 12–18) with data from the Panel Study of Income Dynamics's Child Development Supplement (Keyes 2009), in a national

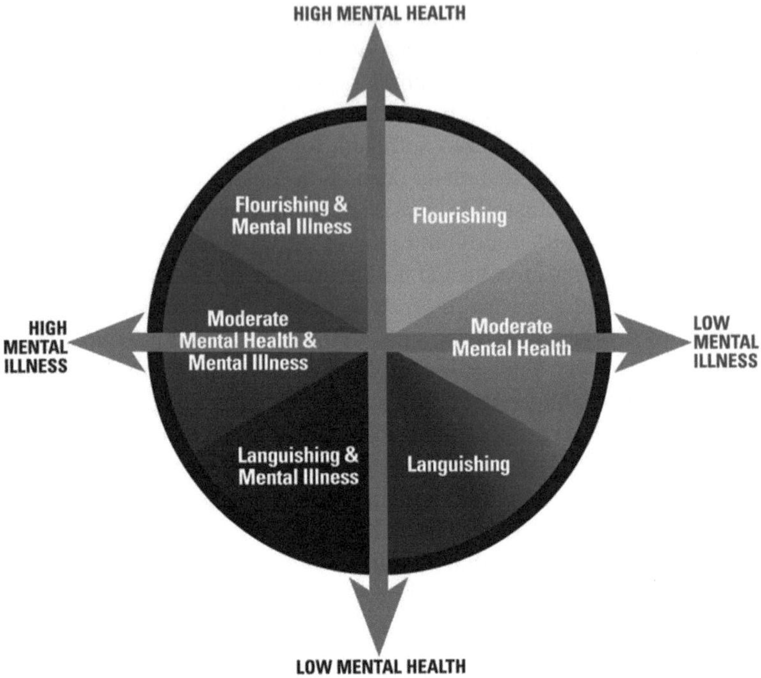

Fig. 1.1 The two continua model

study of Dutch adults (Westerhof and Keyes 2008, 2010) and in Setswana-speaking South African adults using the MHC-SF (Keyes et al. 2008).

Based on the dual continua model shown in Fig. 1.1, individuals can be categorized by their recent mental illness status and according to their level of mental health—whether they have languishing, moderate, or flourishing mental health. One implication of the dual continua model is that the absence of mental illness does not imply the presence of mental health. In the American adult population between 25 and 74 years, just over 75 % were free of three common mental disorders during the past year (i.e., major depressive episode [MDE], panic disorder [PD], and generalized anxiety [GAD]). However, while just over three-quarters were free of mental illness during the past year, only about 20 % were flourishing. A second implication of the dual continua is that the presence of mental illness does not imply the absence of mental health. Of the 23 % of adults with any mental illness, 14.5 % had moderate, and 1.5 % had flourishing mental health. Thus, almost 7 of every 10 adults with a recent mental illness (MDE, panic, or GAD) had moderate or flourishing mental health. While the absence of mental illness does not mean the presence of mental health (i.e., flourishing), the presence of mental illness does not imply the absence of some level of good mental health.

Another important implication of the dual continua model is that the level of mental health should differentiate the level of functioning among individuals free of, and those with, a mental illness. Put differently, anything less than flourishing mental health is associated with impaired functioning both for individuals with and without a mental illness. Findings consistently show that adults and adolescents who are diagnosed as anything less than flourishing are functioning worse in terms of physical health outcomes, health-care utilization, missed days of work, and psychosocial functioning (Keyes 2002, 2005b, 2006, 2007, 2009). Over all outcomes to date, individuals who are flourishing function better (e.g., fewer missed days of work) than those with moderate mental health, who in turn function better than languishing ones—and this is true for both individuals with a recent mental illness and those free of a recent mental illness.

1.3.3 Hygieia: Toward Promotion and Protection of Flourishing

Progress has been slow in bringing mental health promotion and protection (MHPP) into the mainstream of debates about how to address the problem of mental illness. Admittedly, there has been a deficit of scientific evidence supporting the "promotion" and the "protection" axioms of MHPP. Central to the argument behind *promotion* is the hypothesis that gains in level of mental health should decrease the risk of mental illness over time. Central to the argument behind *protection* is the hypothesis that losses of mental health increase the risk of mental illness over time, and therefore efforts should be made to prevent, and to respond to, the loss of good mental health. Findings recently published (Keyes et al. 2010) using the ten-year follow-up of the MIDUS national sample strongly supported the protection and promotion hypotheses.

In 1995 and in the 2005 follow-up of the MIDUS sample, adults completed the long form of the Mental Health Continuum (MHC-LF; Keyes 2002, 2005a) and the Composite International Diagnostic Interview Short Form (CIDI-SF; Kessler et al. 1998). Studies have shown that the CIDI-SF has excellent diagnostic sensitivity and diagnostic specificity as compared with diagnoses based on the full CIDI in the National Comorbidity Study (Kessler et al. 1999). During the telephone interview, the CIDI-SF was used to assess whether respondents exhibited symptoms indicative of major depression episode (MDE), generalized anxiety disorder (GAD), and panic attack (PA) during the past 12 months.

We found that the prevalence of levels of mental health and illness in 1995 and 2005 was similar, suggesting the levels of positive mental health may be stable over time. The prevalence of mental illness was about the same in 1995 (18.5 %) as in 2005 (17.5 %); approximately eight out of every ten adults were free of any mental illness in 1995 and in 2005. The prevalence of any mental illness and the absence of mental illness appear to be stable over time. However, of the 17.5 % with any mental illness in 2005, just over half (52 %) were "new cases" insofar as these adults did not have any of the three mental disorders in 1995. Thus, mental illness is dynamic over time, with about half of the people recovering that is replaced by another half of new cases.

The prevalence of flourishing is 3.2 % higher in 2005, up from 19.2 % in 1995. The prevalence of moderate mental health is 3.7 % lower in 2005, which is down from 64.1 % in 1995. The prevalence of languishing is 0.5 % higher in 2005, slightly up from 16.7 % in 1995. Compared with mental illness, levels of mental health—particularly moderate mental health and flourishing—appear slightly more dynamic at the level of the population. That is, there is a slight decline in moderate and slight increase in flourishing mental health at the population level. Overall, mental health appears to be relatively stable at this level. However, only 45 % of those languishing in 1995 are languishing in 2005; 51 % improved to moderate and 4 % improved to flourishing mental health. Only 51 % of those flourishing in 1995 are flourishing in 2005—46 % declined to moderate and 3 % declined to languishing mental health in 2005. Two-thirds of those with moderate mental health in 1995 had moderate mental health in 2005. Of those with moderate mental health in 1995, about 19 % improved to flourishing, and 14 % declined to languishing, mental health in 2005. Like mental illness, level of mental health is dynamic over time.

1.3.4 Hygieia Validated: Confirmation of the Promotion and Protection Hypotheses

The changes in mental health level were strongly predictive of future mental illness. First, findings supported the protection hypothesis. Those who declined to moderate mental health were nearly four times (adjusted[1] odds ratio [OR] = 3.7) more likely to have a mental illness in 2005 as those who stayed flourishing. Thus, the first loss of good mental health—from flourishing to moderate mental health—results in a rise in the risk of future mental illness. Adults whose mental health stayed at moderate were over four times (OR = 4.4) as likely to have a 2005 mental illness as those who stayed flourishing. Compared to those who stayed at moderate mental health, those who declined to languishing—almost all of whom had moderate mental health in 1995—represented an 86 % increase in the odds ratio of a 2005 mental illness (i.e., $8.2 - 4.4 = 3.2 \div 4.4 = .864$). Thus, protection against the loss of moderate mental health can mitigate the risk of future mental illness.

Findings also supported the promotion hypothesis. Individuals who stayed languishing were over six times (OR = 6.6), while those who improved to moderate mental health were over three times (OR = 3.4) to have a 2005 mental illness. Compared to staying languishing, improving to moderate mental health cuts the risk of future mental illness by nearly half (i.e., $6.6 - 3.4$ $3.2 \div 6.6 = .484$). Individuals who improved to flourishing—most of whom had moderate mental health in 1995—had no more high risk of future mental illness than those who stayed flourishing.

[1]All models controlled for 1995 mental illness, age, sex, race, education, marital status in 2005 and employment status in 2005, and whether respondents had any of 25 physical health conditions in 1995.

Individuals who had any of the three mental illnesses in 1995 were five times (OR = 5.0) more likely than those who stayed flourishing to have one of the same mental illnesses in 2005. Our findings illustrate that the absence of flourishing mental health is as serious a risk factor for future mental illness as those who started with one of the mental illness. Almost half of the study sample who were free of any mental illness in 1995 but had moderate mental health in 2005 (i.e., 7.8 % declined + 35.5 % stayed + 4.7 % improved = 48 % with moderate mental health in 2005) had nearly as high an odds of mental illness in 2005 as the 18.5 % who had a mental illness in 1995. Moreover, one in ten of the study sample was free of any mental illness in 1995 but had languishing mental health in 2005 (i.e., 3.9 % stayed + 6.5 % declined = 10.4 % with languishing in 2005) had a higher odds of mental illness in 2005 than the 18.5 % who had a mental illness in 1995. In short, nearly six in every ten American adults (i.e., 48 % with moderate + 10.4 % with languishing mental health = 58.4 %) otherwise free of MDE, GAD, or PA have about as high or even higher risk of a future mental illness than individuals who had one of those mental disorders to start.

1.4 Conclusion

Ancient civilizations in the West (viz., the Greeks) conceived of health and happiness as ideals, as values, and as one of the highest goods in life (see Sigerist 1941). Well-being was not merely an end; it also was a means to creating and sustaining a good society. Today, mental as well as physical health are considered forms of human capital, because studies consistently link the presence of mental illness and chronic physical disease to high levels of social and economic burden to society, in terms of disability, premature death, and direct and indirect costs. Health, and not solely industriousness or creativity, is now viewed among the greatest sources of the "wealth" of a nation, for it is tied to the growth and development of nations (Berger et al. 2003; Bloom and Canning 2000; Sullivan 2004).

Many scholars and movements, such as positive psychology, lament that too much research on "health" has focused mainly on the presence and absence of disease and illness rather than also the presence and absence of health and well-being (Keyes and Grzywacz 2005). In this chapter, we have argued there is a good reason for the rise of the pathogenic (panacea) focus of nations due to the demographic transition that marks the change in economic development of a nation. At the start, life expectancy is shorter, and the causes of illness and death are acute and infectious. As a nation shifts away from a largely rural and agrarian subsistence to an industrialized and more urban economic system, the nation develops a focus on the causes of disease and death and focuses on the reduction of mortality. As it gains control over the causes of death, fertility remains high, and during this period the population grows. Life expectancy increases, meaning the population is growing larger and aging as well (living longer), and the causes of illness and death shift from mainly acute and infectious to chronic and preventable causes due to lifestyle.

At this point, the economic pressure to sustain health-care systems with a larger and older population exerts greater need to prevent chronic disease and promote greater quality, not merely quantity, of life. In other words, if a nation, after having increased life expectancy, can make the shift toward promoting greater health in addition to life expectancy, it can mitigate chronic conditions and illness by preventing through the promotion of better health as more than the absence of illness. Put simply, as a nation completes the epidemiological transition, there is a need to heighten a focus on salutogenic (hygieia) aspects of health, focusing on better understanding the causes of well-being.

The rising cost of health care and the aging of the US population have made the salutogenic approach more relevant today than ever. However, unlike most European nations that used the recovery from WWII as an opportunity to nationalize health care, the USA remains a highly medicalized system as described through the sociological literature of medicalization reviewed in this chapter. Although WWII did much to jump-start the study of subjective well-being in the USA, the salutogenic approach to mental health in terms of promoting and protecting flourishing remains a work in progress rather a reality at a national level. Nonetheless, well-being has returned to the West precisely because it now encounters the challenges created by successfully going through the demographic transition. In the same way, we believe nations around the globe now undergoing development will need to confront many of the same challenges of how to balance the pathogenic with the salutogenic approaches and how to focus on quantity of life and illness and also make the shift toward quality of life and well-being.

References

Allport, G. (1961). *Pattern and growth in personality*. Oxford: Holt, Rinehart & Winston.

Berger, M. L., Howell, R., Nicholson, S., & Sharda, C. (2003). Investing in healthy human capital. *Journal of Occupational and Environmental Medicine, 45*, 1213–1225.

Bloom, D. E., & Canning, D. (2000). The health and wealth of nations. *Science, 287*, 1207–1209.

Bradburn, N. M. (1969). *The structure of psychological well-being*. Chicago: Aldine.

Bryant, F. B., & Veroff, J. (1982). The structure of psychological well-being: A sociohistorical analysis. *Journal of Personality and Social Psychology, 43*, 653–673.

Cantril, H. (1965). *The pattern of human concerns*. New Brunswick: Rutgers University Press.

Chisholm, D., Sanderson, K., Ayuso-Mateos, J. L., & Saxena, S. (2004). Reducing the global burden of depression: Population-level analysis of intervention cost-effectiveness in 14 world regions. *The British Journal of Psychiatry, 184*, 393–403.

Davis, N. J. (2002). The promotion of mental health and the prevention of mental and behavioral disorders: Surely the time is right. *International Journal of Emergency Mental Health, 4*, 3–29.

Diener, E. (1984). Subjective well-being. *Psychological Bulletin, 95*, 542–575.

Diener, E., Emmons, R. A., Larsen, R. J., & Griffin, S. (1985). The satisfaction with life scale. *Journal of Personality Assessment, 49*, 71–75.

Diener, E., Suh, E. M., Lucas, R. E., & Smith, H. L. (1999). Subjective well-being: Three decades of progress. *Psychological Bulletin, 125*, 276–302.

Erikson, E. H. (1950). *Childhood and society*. New York: Norton.

Erikson, E. H. (1959). Identity and the life cycle. *Psychological Issues, 1*, 18–164.

Gallagher, M. W., Lopez, S. J., & Preacher, K. J. (2009). The hierarchical structure of well-being. *Journal of Personality, 77*, 1025–1049.

Greenspoon, P. J., & Saklofske, D. H. (2001). Toward an integration of subjective well-being and psychopathology. *Social Indicators Research, 54*, 81–108.

Gurin, G., Veroff, J., & Feld, S. (1960). *Americans view their mental health*. New York: Basic Books.

Hart, G. D. (1965). Asclepius: God of medicine. *Canadian Medical Association Journal, 92*(5), 232–236.

Headey, B., Kelley, J., & Wearing, A. (1993). Dimensions of mental health: Life satisfaction, positive affect, anxiety, and depression. *Social Indicators Research, 29*, 63–82.

Health and Welfare Canada. (1988). *Mental health for Canadians: Striking a balance*. Ottawa: Supply and Services Canada.

Huppert, F. A., & Whittington, J. E. (2003). Evidence for the independence of positive and negative well-being: Implications for quality of life assessment. *British Journal of Health Psychology, 8*, 107–122.

Insel, T. R., & Scolnick, E. M. (2006). Cure therapeutics and strategic prevention: Raising the bar for mental health research. *Molecular Psychiatry, 11*, 11–17.

Jahoda, M. (1958). *Current concepts of positive mental health*. New York: Basic Books.

Jané-Llopis, E., Barry, M., Hosman, C., & Patel, V. (2005). What works in mental health promotion. *Promotion & Education, Suppl. 2*, 9–25.

Jung, C. G. (1933). *Modern man in search of a soul* (W. S. Dell & C. F. Baynes, Trans.). New York: Hartcourt, Brace & World.

Kahneman, D., Diener, E., & Schwarz, N. (Eds.). (1999). *Well-being: The foundations of hedonic psychology*. New York: Russell Sage.

Kessler, R. C., Andrews, G., Mroczek, D., Ustun, B., & Wittchen, H.-U. (1998). The world health organization composite international diagnostic interview short form (CIDI–SF). *International Journal of Methods in Psychiatric Research, 7*, 171–185.

Kessler, R. C., DuPont, R. L., Berglund, P., & Wittchen, H.-U. (1999). Impairment in pure and comorbid generalized anxiety disorder and major depression at 12 months in two national surveys. *The American Journal of Psychiatry, 156*, 1915–1923.

Kessler, R. C., Berglund, P., Demler, O., Jin, R., Merikangas, K. R., & Walters, E. E. (2005). Lifetime prevalence and age-of-onset distributions of DSM-IV disorders in the national comorbidity survey replication. *Archives of General Psychiatry, 62*, 593–602.

Keyes, C. L. M. (1998). Social well-being. *Social Psychology Quarterly, 61*, 121–140.

Keyes, C. L. M. (2002). The mental health continuum: From languishing to flourishing in life. *Journal of Health and Social Behavior, 43*, 207–222.

Keyes, C. L. M. (2005a). Mental illness and/or mental health? Investigating axioms of the complete health model. *Journal of Consulting and Clinical Psychology, 73*, 539–548.

Keyes, C. L. M. (2005b). Chronic physical disease and aging: Is mental health a potential protective factor? *Ageing International, 30*, 88–114.

Keyes, C. L. M. (2006). Mental health in adolescence: Is America's youth flourishing? *The American Journal of Orthopsychiatry, 76*, 395–402.

Keyes, C. L. M. (2007). Promoting and protecting mental health as flourishing: A complementary strategy for improving national mental health. *American Psychologist, 62*, 95–108.

Keyes, C. L. M. (2009). The nature and importance of positive mental health in America's adolescents. In R. Gilman, E. S. Huebner, & M. J. Furlong (Eds.), *Handbook of positive psychology in schools* (pp. 9–23). New York: Routledge.

Keyes, C. L. M., & Grzywacz, J. G. (2005). Health as a complete state: The added value in work performance and healthcare costs. *Journal of Environmental and Occupational Health, 47*, 523–532.

Keyes, C. L. M., & Ryff, C. D. (1999). Psychological well-being in midlife. In S. L. Willis & J. D. Reid (Eds.), *Middle aging: Development in the third quarter of life* (pp. 161–180). Orlando: Academic.

Keyes, C. L. M., Shmotkin, D., & Ryff, C. D. (2002). Optimizing well-being: The empirical encounter of two traditions. *Journal of Personality and Social Psychology, 82*, 1007–1022.
Keyes, C. L. M., Wissing, M., Potgieter, J. P., Temane, M., Kruger, A., & van Rooy, S. (2008). Evaluation of the Mental Health Continuum Short Form (MHC-SF) in Setswana speaking South Africans. *Clinical Psychology & Psychotherapy, 15*, 181–192.
Keyes, C. L. M., Dhingra, S. S., & Simoes, E. J. (2010). Change in level of positive mental health as a predictor of future risk of mental illness. *American Journal of Public Health, 100*, 2366–2371.
King, L. A., & Napa, C. K. (1998). What makes a life good? *Journal of Personality and Social Psychology, 75*, 156–165.
Land, K. C. (1975). Social indicators models: An overview. In K. C. Land & S. Spilerman (Eds.), *Social indicator models* (pp. 5–36). New York: Russell Sage.
Lucas, R. E., Diener, E., & Suh, E. (1996). Discriminant validity of well-being measures. *Journal of Personality and Social Psychology, 71*, 616–628.
Martin, J. A., Hamilton, B. E., Sutton, P. D., Ventura, S. J., Mathews, T. J., & Osterman, M. J. K. (2010). *Births: Final data for 2008. National Vital Statistics Report, 59(1)*, 1–72. Retrieved from http://www.cdc.gov/nchs/data/nvsr/nvsr59/nvsr59_01.pdf
Maslow, A. (1968). *Toward a psychology of being* (2nd ed.). New York: Van Nostrand.
Masse, R., Poulin, C., Dassa, C., Lambert, J., Belair, S., & Battaglini, A. (1998). The structure of mental health higher-order confirmatory factor analyses of psychological distress and wellbeing measures. *Social Indicators Research, 45*, 475–504.
McKinlay, J. B., & McKinlay, S. J. (1977). The questionable effect of medical measures on the decline of mortality in the United States in the twentieth century. *The Milbank Memorial Fund Quarterly, 55*, 405–428.
Murray, C. J. L., & Lopez, A. D. (Eds.). (1996). *The global burden of disease: A comprehensive assessment of mortality and disability from diseases, injuries, and risk factors in 1990 and projected to 2020*. Cambridge, MA: Harvard School of Public Health.
Numbers, R. (2001). Fall and rise of the American medical profession. In J. H. Warner & J. Tighe (Eds.), *Major problems in the history of American medicine and public health* (pp. 298–303). Boston: Houghton Mifflin.
Omran, A. R. (1971). The epidemiologic transition: A theory of the epidemiology of population change. *The Milbank Memorial Fund Quarterly, 49*(4), 509–538.
Porter, R. (2002). *Blood and guts: A short history of medicine*. New York: W.W. Norton and Company.
Robitschek, C., & Keyes, C. L. M. (2009). The structure of Keyes' model of mental health and the role of personal growth initiative as a parsimonious predictor. *Journal of Counseling Psychology, 56*, 321–329.
Rogers, C. R. (1961). *On becoming a person*. Boston: Houghton Mifflin.
Rothman, D. J., Marcus, S., & Kiceluk, S. A. (Eds.). (1995). *Medicine and western civilization*. New Brunswick: Rutgers University Press.
Ryan, R. M., & Deci, E. L. (2001). On happiness and human potentials: A review of research on hedonic and eudaimonic well-being. *Annual Review of Psychology, 52*, 141–166.
Ryff, C. D. (1989). Happiness is everything, or is it? Explorations on the meaning of psychological well–being. *Journal of Personality and Social Psychology, 57*, 1069–1081.
Ryff, C. D., & Keyes, C. L. M. (1995). The structure of psychological well-being revisited. *Journal of Personality and Social Psychology, 69*, 719–727.
Secker, J. (1998). Current conceptualizations of mental health and mental health promotion. *Health Education Research, 13*, 57–66.
Severin, F. T. (1965). *Humanistic viewpoints in psychology*. New York: McGraw-Hill.
Shmotkin, D. (1998). Declarative and differential aspects of subjective well-being and implications for mental health in later life. In J. Lomranz (Ed.), *Handbook of aging and mental health: An integrative approach* (pp. 15–43). New York: Plenum.
Sigerist, H. E. (1941). *Medicine and human welfare*. New Haven: Yale University Press.
Smith, M. B. (1959). Research strategies toward a conception of positive mental health. *American Psychologist, 14*, 673–681.

Starr, P. (1982). *Social transformation of American medicine*. New York: Basic Books.
Suldo, S. M., & Shaffer, E. J. (2008). Looking beyond psychopathology: The dual-factor model of mental health in youth. *School Psychology Review, 37*, 52–68.
Sullivan, S. (2004). Making the business case for health and productivity management. *Journal of Occupational and Environmental Medicine, 46*, 56–61.
Ustun, T. B. (1999). The global burden of mental disorders. *American Journal of Public Health, 89*, 1315–1318.
Ustun, T. B., Ayuso-Mateos, J. L., Chatterji, S., Mathers, C. D., & Murray, C. J. L. (2004). Global burden of depressive disorders in the year 2000. *The British Journal of Psychiatry, 184*, 386–392.
Veit, C. T., & Ware, J. E. (1983). The structure of psychological distress and well-being in general populations. *Journal of Consulting and Clinical Psychology, 51*, 730–742.
Waterman, A. S. (1990). The relevance of Aristotle's conception of eudaimonia for the psychological study of happiness. *Theoretical and Philosophical Psychology, 10*, 39–44.
Waterman, A. S. (1993). Two conceptions of happiness: Contrasts of personal expressiveness (eudaimonia) and hedonic enjoyment. *Journal of Personality and Social Psychology, 64*, 678–691.
Watson, D., & Clark, L. A. (1997). Measurement and mismeasurement of mood: Recurrent and emergent issues. *Journal of Personality Assessment, 68*, 267–296.
Weber, M. (1947). *The theory of social and economic organization*. (A. M. Henderson & T. Parsons, Trans.). New York: The Free Press.
Weitz, R. (2010). *The sociology of health, illness, and health care: A critical approach*. Boston: Wadsworth Cengage Learning.
Westerhof, G. J., & Keyes, C. L. M. (2008). Mental health is more than the absence of mental illness. *Monthly Mental Health* (In Dutch, Summary in English), *63*, 808–820.
Westerhof, G. J., & Keyes, C. L. M. (2010). Mental illness and mental health: The two continua model across the lifespan. *Journal of Adult Development, 17*, 110–119.
World Health Organization. (2004). *Promoting mental health: Concepts, emerging evidence, practice* (Summary report). Geneva: Author.

Chapter 2
The Psychosomatic View

Nicoletta Sonino and Giovanni A. Fava

2.1 Introduction

The ongoing progress in scientific medicine and technology in recent years has led to further splitting of knowledge and consequent fragmentation in the response to health issues. On the other hand, this is in contrast with research evidence that points to the importance of incorporating psychosocial aspects and holistic view in the approach to the person presenting with any health problem. While nothing is changing in clinical practice modalities of dealing with different phases of disease management, there is a clear need to improve patient-physician relationships, patient satisfaction and compliance, and final outcomes.

The interdisciplinary field of psychosomatic medicine has the potential to fill this gap providing both the cognitive frame of reference and the practical tools that can be employed in everyday clinical practice.

2.2 History and Current Developments

The term "psychosomatic" entails different meanings and connotations, which may explain its varying degrees of popularity. Heinroth introduced the concept in 1818, but modern psychosomatic medicine developed in the first half of the past century.

N. Sonino (✉)
Department of Statistical Sciences, University of Padova, Padua, Italy

Department of Psychiatry, State University of New York at Buffalo, Buffalo, NY, USA
e-mail: nicoletta.sonino@unipd.it

G.A. Fava
Department of Psychiatry, State University of New York at Buffalo, Buffalo, NY, USA

Department of Psychology, University of Bologna, Bologna, Italy

A. Morandi and A.N. Narayanan Nambi (eds.), *An Integrated View of Health and Well-being*, Cross-Cultural Advancements in Positive Psychology 5, DOI 10.1007/978-94-007-6689-1_2,

It resulted from the interaction of different concepts having an ancient tradition in Western medicine: psychogenesis of disease and holism (Lipowski 1986). The idea of psychogenesis characterized the first phase of development of psychosomatic medicine (1930–1960) and evolved toward the definition of "psychosomatic disease" for a number of conditions in which psychological aspects seemed to have a preponderant role. Despite early criticism, the psychogenic postulate continued to exert explanatory power in the search for pathogenetic mechanisms. For example, a physical illness such as peptic ulcer was believed to be caused by psychological factors.

The term "psychosomatic disorder" was strongly criticized by several psychosomatic researchers, including Kissen (1963), Engel (1967), and Lipowski (1986). Kissen (1963) provided a better specification of the term "psychosomatic." He clarified that the relative weight of psychosocial factors may vary from one individual to another within the same illness and underscored the basic conceptual flaw of considering diseases as homogeneous entities. Engel (1967) wrote that the term "psychosomatic disorder" was misleading, since it implied a special class of disorders of psychogenic aetiology and, by inference, the absence of a psychosomatic interface in other diseases. On the other hand, he viewed reductionism that overlooked the impact of non-biological circumstances upon biological processes as a major cause of mistreatment. Lipowski (1986) criticized the concept of psychosomatic disorder since it tended to perpetuate the obsolete notion of psychogenesis, which is incompatible with the doctrine of multi-causality, a core postulate of current psychosomatic medicine. With his work, he gave an invaluable contribution in setting the scope, mission, and methods of psychosomatic medicine.

Among major innovations stands the introduction of the biopsychosocial model of illness by Engel (1977). It allows illness to be viewed as a result of interacting mechanisms at the cellular, tissue, organismic, interpersonal, and environmental levels. Accordingly, the study of every disease must include the individual, his body, and his surrounding environment as essential components of the total system (Novack et al. 2007). This model retains today its full impact in clinical research and practice (Fava and Sonino 2008).

An updated definition of psychosomatic medicine and its boundaries with related disciplines (Fava and Sonino 2010) are illustrated in Box 2.1.

Box 2.1 Psychosomatic Medicine

Definition

Psychosomatic medicine may be defined as a comprehensive, interdisciplinary framework for:

(a) Assessment of psychosocial factors affecting individual vulnerability, course, and outcome of any type of disease
(b) Holistic consideration of patient care in clinical practice
(c) Integration of psychological therapies in the prevention, treatment, and rehabilitation of medical disease

(continued)

Box 2.1 (continued)

Boundaries

In the USA, psychosomatic medicine has recently become a subspecialty recognized by the American Board of Medical Specialties. This may lead to identifying psychosomatic medicine with consultation-liaison psychiatry (Gitlin et al. 2004). Consultation-liaison psychiatry is clearly within the field of psychiatry; its setting is the medical or surgical clinic or ward, and its focus is the comorbid states of patients with medical disorders (Wise 2000). Psychosomatic medicine is, by definition, multidisciplinary. It is not confined to psychiatry but may concern any field of medicine. Not surprisingly, in countries such as Germany and Japan, psychosomatic activities have achieved an independent status (Deter 2004).

Subdisciplines

The general psychosomatic approach has resulted in a number of subdisciplines within their own areas of application: psychooncology, psychonephrology, psychoneuroendocrinology, psychoimmunology, psychodermatology, and others. Such subdisciplines have developed clinical services, scientific societies, and medical journals.

2.3 Psychosocial Factors and Individual Vulnerability

It has become increasingly clear that we can improve medical care by paying more attention to psychological aspects of medical assessment (Kroenke 2002; Fava et al. 2012), with particular reference to the role of stress (McEwen 2007; Fava et al. 2010). A number of factors have been implied to modulate individual vulnerability to disease.

2.3.1 Stressful Life Events

The role of early developmental factors in susceptibility to disease has been a frequent object of psychosomatic investigation (McEwen 2007; Romans and Cohen 2008). Using animal models, events such as premature separation from the mother have consistently resulted in pathophysiological modifications, such as increased hypothalamic-pituitary-adrenal axis (HPA) activation (McEwen 2007). They may render the human individual more vulnerable to the effects of stress later in life. There has been also considerable interest in the association of childhood physical and sexual abuse with medical disorders later in life. This link has been postulated for chronic pain and irritable bowel syndrome and several adverse health outcomes (functional disability and risk behaviors), yet the evidence currently available does not allow any firm conclusion (Romans and Cohen 2008).

The notion that events and situations in a person's life, which are meaningful to him or her, may be followed by ill health has been a common clinical observation. The introduction of structured methods of data collection and control groups has allowed to substantiate the link between life events in the year preceding the onset of symptoms and a number of medical disorders, encompassing endocrine, cardiovascular, respiratory, gastrointestinal, autoimmune, skin, and neoplastic disease (Novack et al. 2007; Theorell 2012).

2.3.2 Chronic Stress and Allostatic Load

Subtle and long-standing life situations should not too readily be dismissed as minor and negligible, since chronic, daily life stresses may be experienced by the individual as taxing or exceeding his or her coping skills. McEwen (2007) proposed a formulation of the relationship between stress and the processes leading to disease based on the concept of allostasis, the ability of the organism to achieve stability through change. Allostatic load reflects the cumulative effects of stressful experiences in daily life. When the cost of chronic exposure to fluctuating and heightened neural or neuroendocrine responses exceeds the coping resources of an individual, allostatic overload ensues (Fava et al. 2010). Allostatic overload can be assessed on clinical grounds. Biological parameters of allostatic load, such as glycosylated proteins, coagulation/fibrinolysis, and hormonal markers, have been linked to cognitive and physical functioning and mortality (McEwen 2007).

2.3.3 Health Attitudes

Unhealthy lifestyle is a recognized risk factor for most prevalent diseases, such as diabetes, obesity, and cardiovascular illness (Tomba 2012). In 1985, Geoffrey Rose showed that the risk factors for health are almost always normally distributed and supported a general population approach to prevention, instead of targeting those at the highest risk. Accordingly, switching the general population to healthy lifestyles would be a major source of prevention.

2.3.4 Personality and Psychological Well-Being

The notion that personality variables can affect vulnerability to specific diseases was prevalent in the first phase of development of psychosomatic medicine (1930–1960) and was particularly influenced by psychoanalytic investigators, who believed that specific personality profiles underlay specific "psychosomatic diseases." This hypothesis was not supported by subsequent research (Lipowski 1986). Two personality constructs that can potentially affect general vulnerability to disease, type A behavior and alexithymia (i.e., the inability to express emotion), have attracted considerable attention, but their relationship with health is still controversial (Cosci 2012). However, personality variables (e.g., obsessive-compulsive, paranoid, impulsive) may deeply affect how a patient views illness, what it means to him/her, and his/her interactions with others, including medical staff.

Positive health is often regarded as the absence of illness, despite the fact that, half a century ago, the World Health Organization defined health as a "state of complete physical, mental, and social well-being and not merely the absence of disease or infirmity" (further discussion of this issue can be found in Chaps. 1 and 9 of this volume). Research on psychological well-being has indicated that it derives from the interaction of several related dimensions (Ryff and Singer 1996; Fava and Tomba 2009). Several studies have suggested that psychological well-being plays a buffering role in coping with stress and has a favorable impact on disease course (Pressman and Cohen 2005).

2.3.5 Social Support

Prospective population studies have substantiated the role of social support in relation to mortality, psychiatric and physical morbidity, and recovery and adjustment to chronic disease (Fava and Sonino 2010). An area that is now called "social neuroscience" is beginning to address the effects of the environment and social network on the brain and the physiology it regulates (McEwen 2007).

2.3.6 Spirituality

Religiosity and spirituality (broadly defined as any feelings, thoughts, experiences, and behaviors that arise from the search for the "sacred") have been a matter of growing interest in epidemiological research (Chida et al. 2009). Religiosity appeared to have a favorable effect on survival, that is, independent from behavioral factors (smoking, drinking, etc.), negative affect, and degree of social support. This topic is also addressed in Chap. 9, as well as in the chapters included in Part II of this volume, since attention to the spiritual dimension is an integral part of the Āyurveda approach to health.

2.4 Need for Holistic Consideration in Patient Care

Psychosocial and biological factors interact in a number of ways in the course of medical disease. Their varying influence together with each individual response determines the unique quality of the experience and attitude of every patient in any given episode of illness.

2.4.1 Psychiatric Disturbances

Psychiatric illness appears to be strongly associated with medical diseases. Mental disorders increase the risk for communicable and noncommunicable diseases; many health conditions increase the risk for mental disturbances; comorbidity complicates recognition and treatment of medical disorders (Prince et al. 2007).

There is evidence that psychiatric disturbances in the course of medical disease are substantially different from those which can be found in psychiatric settings in terms of clinical characteristics, prognosis, and response to treatment.

Major depression has emerged as an extremely important source of comorbidity in medical disorders (Katon 2003). It was found to affect quality of life and social functioning and lead to increased health care utilization, to be associated with higher mortality, particularly in the elderly, to have an impact on compliance, and to increase susceptibility to medical illness.

2.4.2 Psychological Disturbances

Current emphasis in psychiatry is about assessment of symptoms resulting in syndromes identified by diagnostic criteria (DSM). However, there is emerging awareness that also psychological symptoms which do not reach the threshold of a psychiatric disorder may affect quality of life and entail pathophysiological and therapeutic implications. This has led to the development of Diagnostic Criteria for Psychosomatic Research (DCPR) (Box 2.2) and a specific interview to assess patients (see examples in Box 2.3). The DCPR were introduced in 1995 and tested in various clinical settings (Porcelli and Sonino 2007).

Box 2.2 The Diagnostic Criteria for Psychosomatic Research (DCPR)

1. Health anxiety
2. Thanatophobia
3. Disease phobia
4. Illness denial
5. Persistent somatization
6. Conversion symptoms
7. Functional somatic symptoms secondary to a psychiatric disorder
8. Anniversary reaction
9. Demoralization
10. Irritable mood
11. Type A behavior
12. Alexithymia

The advantage of this classification is that it departs from the dichotomy between organic and functional and from the misleading and dangerous assumption that if organic factors cannot be identified, there should be psychiatric reasons which may be able to fully explain the somatic symptomatology. The psychosomatic literature provides an endless series of examples where psychological factors could only account for part of the unexplained medical disorder (Fava et al. 2012). Similarly, the presence of an established medical disorder does not exclude but indeed increases the likelihood of psychological distress and abnormal illness behavior (Fava and Sonino 2010).

Box 2.3 Examples of Questions Derived from the Diagnostic Criteria for Psychosomatic Research (DCPR)

Demoralization

Do you feel you have failed to meet your expectations or those of other people?
Is there an urgent problem you feel unable to cope with?
Do you experience feelings of helplessness, hopelessness, and/or giving up?

Irritable Mood

When you feel irritable, do you need to make an increased effort to control your temper?
Do you have uncontrollable verbal or behavioral outbursts?

Illness Denial

Have you ever neglected to bring to your physician's attention serious symptoms or ignored your physician's diagnosis and recommendations?
If the physician tells you that you have a disease and prescribe you drugs, a diet, or physical activity, do you follow the medical advice?

2.4.3 *Quality of Life*

While there is neither a precise nor an agreed definition of quality of life, research in this area seeks essentially two kinds of information: the functional status of the individual and the patient's appraisal of health. Indeed, the subjective perception of health status (e.g., lack of well-being, demoralization, and difficulties fulfilling personal and family responsibilities) is as valid as that of the clinician in evaluating outcome (Fava and Sonino 2010). This is an aspect that deserves more attention in clinical assessments.

2.5 Integration of Psychological Interventions in Medicine

Psychological interventions in the medically ill may be performed by different health professionals and may range from reassurance and effective communication to specific psychotherapeutic and psychopharmacological treatments.

2.5.1 *Treatment of Psychiatric Comorbidity*

Psychiatric disorders are frequently unrecognized and untreated in medical settings, with widespread harmful consequences for the individual and the society (Prince et al. 2007). Treatment of psychiatric comorbidity such as depression, with either pharmacological or psychotherapeutic interventions, markedly improves health-related functioning and the quality of life, although an effect on medical outcome has not been demonstrated.

2.5.2 *Psychosocial Interventions*

The use of psychotherapeutic strategies (cognitive-behavioral therapy, stress management procedures, brief dynamic therapy) in controlled investigations has yielded a substantial improvement in a number of medical disorders (Kaupp et al. 2005). Examples are interventions that increase social support and enhance coping capacity in patients with breast cancer and malignant melanoma or employ writing about personal stressful experiences in asthma and rheumatoid arthritis (see Chap. 9 for further details on this issue).

Research on psychotherapy has disclosed common therapeutic ingredients relevant to any physician-patient relationship, listed in Box 2.4 (Fava and Sonino 2010).

Box 2.4 Nonspecific Therapeutic Ingredients

The therapist's full availability for specific times	= *Attention*
The patient's opportunity to ventilate thoughts and feelings	= *Disclosure*
An emotionally charged, confiding relationship with a helping person	= *High arousal*
A plausible explanation of the symptoms	= *Interpretation*
The active participation of patient and therapist in a ritual or procedure that is believed by both to be the means of restoring the patient's health	= *Rituals*

Abnormal illness behavior may greatly benefit from this type of intervention. For many years, abnormal illness behavior has been viewed mainly as an expression of personality predisposition and considered to be refractory to psychotherapy. There is now evidence to challenge such pessimistic stance. For instance, several controlled studies indicate that hypochondriasis is a treatable condition by the use of simple cognitive strategies (Fava and Sonino 2010).

Lifestyle Modification

A basic psychosomatic assumption is the consideration of patients as partners in managing disease. The partnership paradigm includes both collaborative care, a patient-physician relationship in which physicians and patients make health decisions together (Joosten et al. 2008), and self-management, a plan that provides patients with problem-solving skills to enhance their self-efficacy (Bodenheimer et al. 2002). The benefits of modifying lifestyle have been particularly demonstrated in coronary heart disease (Rozanski et al. 1999) and type 2 diabetes (Sperl-Hillen et al. 2011; Sonino et al. 2007). As elucidated in Part II and in Chap. 9 of this volume, attention to lifestyle is one of the pillars of Āyurveda. Further, psychological treatments may be effective in health-damaging behaviors, such as smoking (Tomba 2012).

2.6 Current Issues

There have been major transformations in health care needs in the past decades. Chronic disease is now the principal cause of disability, and use of health services consumes almost 80 % of health expenditures (Bodenheimer et al. 2002). Current health care is still conceptualized in terms of acute care perceived as a product processing, where the patients is a customer, who can, at best, select among the services that are offered. Yet, as Hart (1995) has pointed out, in health care the product is clearly health and the patients is one of the producers, not just a customer. As a result, "optimally efficient health production depends on a general shift of patients from their traditional roles as passive or adversarial consumers, to become producers of health jointly with their health professionals" (Hart 1995, p. 383).

The need to include consideration of function in daily life, productivity, performance of social roles, intellectual capacity, emotional stability, and well-being has emerged as a crucial part of clinical investigation and patient care. Patients have become increasingly aware of these issues. The commercial success of books on complementary medicine and positive practices as well as the upsurge of mind-body medicine exemplify the receptivity of the general public to messages of well-being pursuit. Psychosomatic interventions may respond to these emerging needs within the established medical system and may play an important role in supporting the healing process.

Medically unexplained symptoms are common in medical patients and increase medical utilization and costs (Hatcher and Arroll 2008). The traditional medical specialties, based mostly on organ systems (e.g., cardiology, gastroenterology), appear to be more and more inadequate in dealing with symptoms and problems which cut across organ system subdivisions and require a holistic approach. The interdisciplinary dimension that characterizes most rehabilitation units and pain clinics exemplifies this concept.

The benefits of modifying lifestyle by population-based measures are increasingly demonstrated (Fava and Sonino 2010; Sperl-Hillen et al. 2011; Tomba 2012). Yet, at present almost all of health care spending is directed at biomedically oriented care. Overemphasis on pharmacological treatment has led to a dangerous reductionism and overlooks the fact that therapeutic outcomes are the result of several ingredients, which may be specific or nonspecific, as outlined above. As Kroenke (2002) argued, neither chronic medical nor psychiatric disorder can be managed adequately in the current environment of general practice, where the typical patient must be seen in 10–15 min or less.

In clinical medicine, there is the tendency to rely exclusively on "hard data," preferably expressed in terms of laboratory results, excluding "soft information" such as impairments and well-being. This soft information can be, however, reliably assessed by clinical rating scales and indexes which have been validated and used in psychosomatic research and practice (Fava et al. 2012). Box 2.5 illustrates how "hard data" and "soft information" need to be incorporated in clinical encounters. It is not that certain disorders lack an explanation; it is our assessment that is mostly inadequate, since it does not incorporate a global psychosomatic approach (Sonino and Peruzzi 2009; Fava et al. 2012). Similarly, within a biopsychosocial model, addressing the origins of disparities in physical and mental health care early in life may produce greater effects than attempting to modify health-related behaviors later or to improve access to health care in adulthood (Shonkoff et al. 2009).

Box 2.5 This Case Illustrates How the Psychosomatic Consideration of a Patient's Complaints May Lead to Better Assessment and Management

A 54-year-old woman was diagnosed with hypothyroidism. She was prescribed thyroid substitution which restored thyroid hormone levels within the normal range but kept feeling miserable, with a very bothersome globus in the throat. She consulted several endocrinologists, who all stated that her thyroid replacement was fine and there was nothing wrong with her, which made her angry and dissatisfied. She was then referred to a psychoneuroendocrinology service. Careful interviewing disclosed the presence of agoraphobia (fear of public spaces and going out alone) with sporadic panic attacks and that she attributed the globus and panic to the thyroid, adjusting herself to thyroid replacement in relation to her current feelings. She also reported marital problems. The psychosomatic assessment and physical examination led to explaining that agoraphobia is a psychological disorder, her globus was related to it, not to the thyroid, and that changing herself thyroid replacement could only make things worse. A brief course of cognitive-behavioral treatment by a psychologist did improve her agoraphobia and marital problems greatly, with disappearance of panic attacks. Only sporadic symptoms of globus related to anxiety persisted.

In conclusion, appraisal of the multifactorial determinants of the cure process may restore a trusting patient-doctor interaction, improving final outcomes. In the late 1970s, a prominent psychosomatic investigator, Morton Reiser (1979), anticipated the success of oriental medical theory and practice in the Western world and identified psychosomatic medicine as the most suitable meeting ground for the two models. Indeed, the psychosomatic research background has consolidated over the past decades in dealing with complex biopsychosocial phenomena and may now provide new effective modalities of patient care.

References

Bodenheimer, T., Lorig, K., Holman, H., & Grumbach, K. (2002). Patient self-management of chronic disease in primary care. *Journal of the American Medical Association, 288*, 2469–2475.

Chida, Y., Steptoe, A., & Powell, L. H. (2009). Religiosity/spirituality and mortality. *Psychotherapy and Psychosomatics, 78*, 81–90.

Cosci, F. (2012). Assessment of personality in psychosomatic medicine: Current concepts. *Advances in Psychosomatic Medicine, 32*, 133–159.

Deter, H. C. (2004). Psychosomatic medicine and psychotherapy. *Advances in Psychosomatic Medicine, 26*, 181–189.

Engel, G. L. (1967). The concept of psychosomatic disorder. *Journal of Psychosomatic Research, 11*, 3–9.

Engel, G. L. (1977). The need for a new medical model: A challenge for biomedicine. *Science, 196*, 129–136.

Fava, G. A., & Sonino, N. (2008). The biopsychosocial model thirty years later. *Psychotherapy and Psychosomatics, 77*, 1–2.

Fava, G. A., & Sonino, N. (2010). Psychosomatic medicine. *International Journal of Clinical Practice, 64*, 1155–1161.

Fava, G. A., & Tomba, E. (2009). Increasing psychological well-being and resilience by psychotherapeutic methods. *Journal of Personality, 77*, 1903–1934.

Fava, G. A., Guidi, J., Semprini, F., Tomba, E., & Sonino, N. (2010). Clinical assessment of allostatic load and clinimetric criteria. *Psychotherapy and Psychosomatics, 79*, 280–284.

Fava, G. A., Sonino, N., & Wise, T. N. (Eds.). (2012). *The psychosomatic assessment. Strategies to improve clinical practice*. Basel: Karger.

Gitlin, D. F., Levenson, J. L., & Lyketsos, C. G. (2004). Psychosomatic medicine: A new psychiatric subspecialty. *Academic Psychiatry, 28*, 4–11.

Hart, J. T. (1995). Clinical and economic consequences of patients as producers. *Journal of Public Health Medicine, 17*, 383–386.

Hatcher, S., & Arroll, B. (2008). Assessment and management of medically unexplained symptoms. *British Medical Journal, 336*, 1124–1128.

Joosten, E. A., DeFuentes-Merillas, L., de Weert, G. H., Sensky, T., van der Staak, C. P., & de Jong, C. A. (2008). Systematic review of the effects of shared decision-making on patient satisfaction, treatment adherence and health status. *Psychotherapy and Psychosomatics, 77*, 219–226.

Katon, W. J. (2003). Clinical and health services relationships between major depression, depressive symptoms and general medical illness. *Biological Psychiatry, 54*, 216–226.

Kaupp, J. W., Rapaport-Hubschman, N., & Spiegel, D. (2005). Psychosocial treatments. In J. L. Levenson (Ed.), *Textbook of psychosomatic medicine* (pp. 923–956). Washington, DC: American Psychiatric Press.

Kissen, D. M. (1963). The significance of syndrome shift and late syndrome association in psychosomatic medicine. *The Journal of Nervous and Mental Disease, 136*, 34–42.

Kroenke, K. (2002). Psychological medicine. *British Medical Journal, 324*, 1536–1537.

Lipowski, Z. J. (1986). Psychosomatic medicine: Past and present. *Canadian Journal of Psychiatry, 31*, 2–21.

McEwen, B. S. (2007). Physiology and neurobiology of stress and adaptation: Central role of the brain. *Physiological Reviews, 87*, 873–904.

Novack, D. H., Cameron, O., Epel, E., Ader, R., Waldstein, S. R., Levenstein, S., Antoni, M. H., & Wainer, A. R. (2007). Psychosomatic medicine: The scientific foundation of the biopsychosocial model. *Academic Psychiatry, 31*, 388–401.

Porcelli, P., & Sonino, N. (Eds.). (2007). *Psychological factors affecting medical conditions*. Basel: Karger.
Pressman, S. D., & Cohen, S. (2005). Does positive affect influence health? *Psychological Bulletin, 131*, 925–971.
Prince, M., Patel, V., Saxena, S., Maj, M., Maselko, J., Phillips, M. R., & Rahman, A. (2007). No health without mental health. *Lancet, 370*, 859–877.
Reiser, M. F. (1979). Psychosomatic medicine: A meeting ground for oriental and occidental medicine theory and practice. *Psychotherapy and Psychosomatics, 31*, 315–323.
Romans, S., & Cohen, M. (2008). Unexplained and underpowered: The relationship between psychosomatic disorders and interpersonal abuse. *Harvard Review of Psychiatry, 16*, 35–44.
Rose, G. (1985). Sick individuals and sick populations. *International Journal of Epidemiology, 14*, 32–38.
Rozanski, A., Blumenthal, J. A., & Kaplan, J. (1999). Impact of psychological factors on the pathogenesis of cardiovascular disease and implications for therapy. *Circulation, 99*, 2192–2217.
Ryff, C. D., & Singer, B. (1996). Psychological well-being. *Psychotherapy and Psychosomatics, 65*, 14–23.
Shonkoff, J. P., Boyce, W. T., & McEwen, B. S. (2009). Neuroscience, molecular biology and the childhood roots of health disparities. *Journal of the American Medical Association, 301*, 2252–2259.
Sonino, N., & Peruzzi, P. (2009). A psychoneuroendocrinology service. *Psychotherapy and Psychosomatics, 78*, 346–351.
Sonino, N., Tomba, E., & Fava, G. A. (2007). Psychosocial approach to endocrine disease. *Advances in Psychosomatic Medicine, 28*, 21–33.
Sperl-Hillen, J., Beaton, S., Fernandes, O., von Worley, A., Vazquez-Benitez, G., Parker, E., Hanson, A., Lavin-Thompkins, J., Glasrud, P., Davis, H., Adams, K., Parsons, W., & Spain, V. (2011). Comparative effectiveness of patient education methods for type 2 diabetes. *Archives of Internal Medicine, 171*, 2001–2010.
Theorell, T. (2012). Evaluating life events and chronic stressors in relation to health. *Advances in Psychosomatic Medicine, 32*, 58–71.
Tomba, E. (2012). Assessment of lifestyle in relation to health. *Advances in Psychosomatic Medicine, 32*, 72–96.
Wise, T. N. (2000). Consultation liaison psychiatry and psychosomatics: Strange bedfellows. *Psychotherapy and Psychosomatics, 69*, 181–183.

Part II
Health and Well-Being in Indian Traditions

Chapter 3
The Perspectives on Reality in Indian Traditions and Their Implications for Health and Well-Being

Kiran Kumar K. Salagame

3.1 Introduction

Health and well-being are often used together as an alliterative phrase, as in kith and kin, to emphasize the positive state in human beings. Sometimes they are used interchangeably, but they have different connotations. In recent times, two different disciplines, viz. health psychology (Dimatteo and Martin 2007) and positive psychology (Sheldon et al. 2011), have claimed health and well-being as their primary subject matter, respectively. Though both are related, health and well-being seem to vary independently. Brief et al. (1993) found people with poor health having high subjective well-being and people with few objective health problems who had low subjective well-being.

Central to the understanding of health and well-being is the famous Cartesian duality between mind and body. Since Western intellectual tradition treated them as separate for the past three centuries, modern medicine being a product of this tradition has become primarily *body centred*. The notions of illness and health including the so-called mental health have developed with a biological orientation. All the efforts in treating illness or in promoting health have our physical body as the focus resulting in trillion-dollar health-care industry globally. Thus we have pharmaceutical industries, development of biomedical technologies and establishment of diagnostic centres, private hospitals, medical education, research facilities and medical insurance companies (see also Chap. 1 for detailed discussion on Western health system and its origins). All these elaborate paraphernalia often focus on aetiology, symptomatology, pathology, epidemiology, diagnostics and treatment of illness, and one is often left to wonder whether it is illness care or health care.

K.K.K. Salagame (✉)
Department of Studies in Psychology, University of Mysore, Mysore, India
e-mail: kikusk@dataone.in; kikusk@gmail.com

A. Morandi and A.N. Narayanan Nambi (eds.), *An Integrated View of Health and Well-being*, Cross-Cultural Advancements in Positive Psychology 5, DOI 10.1007/978-94-007-6689-1_3,

Though these developments are not to be condemned or belittled, there is a flop side of health-care industry. People are finding it difficult to afford the increasing cost of modern health-care system. An article published in *Chicago Tribune* a few years ago (*Chicago Tribune*, 8 August 2007) carries the story of an American who chose to bring his aged parents to Pondicherry, in India, because he found out that the health care is cheaper there than back home. Not only that, many more persons from different countries have been finding that medical care and attention is more sophisticated and technologically advanced in India but less expensive compared to their own countries. However, for a vast majority of Indians, medical care is getting really more expensive and unaffordable due to the increased corporate culture surrounding such services.

I am reminded of an old saying in Sanskrit which reads thus: *vaidyarāja namasthubhyam yamarāajahsahodarah*| *yamastu haratihprānān vaidyah prānān dhanāni ca*|| (Oh doctor, brother of Yama the Lord of death, salutations to you! Yama only snatches life, whereas you take away both life and money!!). This ancient humour probably is more apt in contemporary period, than any other time, when so much money is involved in health enterprise.

The economic factors have been influencing even the illness that one can or cannot afford to have and get treated. I remember here an amusing, yet instructive, TV advertisement of an insurance company. A patient visits a clinic, and the doctor after having examined the chest X-ray says he has a problem with his respiratory system, for which the patient reacts with chagrin, 'it could not be so' and says 'a kidney problem is OK', because insurance company pays for that not for a chest disease! Thus, contemporary health-care practices have become *artha pradhāna* (money or wealth predominant) than *dharma pradhāna* (moral or ethical predominant), though Hippocratic oath continues to be administered to the new graduates!

Definitions of well-being are also loaded with economic considerations. The clinical psychologist Paul Watchel (1989) notes that when gross national product (GNP) is taken as a measure of well-being, even 'the medical costs due to the diseases caused by pollution are figured into the GNP as *pluses* … if less pollution occurred, and as a result less medical treatment was required, this would show up as a drop in the GNP![1]' (p. 88). It is what happens when the materialistic and economic orientation is stretched to its logical limits.

There is a difference between the popular use of the term 'well-being', which usually relates to health and the philosophical use of this term that is broader, but related, and is concerned with the notion of a good life of which health is an aspect (http://plato.stanford.edu/entries/well-being/). Hence, well-being is more related to overall quality of one's life, and economists and sociologists have attempted to pin down the essential objective conditions required for a better quality of life. While social scientists – economists, political scientists and sociologists – have focused on the objective criteria, psychologists have looked into the subjective evaluation of one's level of satisfaction with one's life as the criteria for well-being

---

[1] '!' added for emphasis.

(Diener 1984; Hoorn 2007; Conceição and Bandura 2013). Diener and Seligman (2004) found that mental disorders are a major cause of low well-being and poor mental health almost always causes poor well-being. It is likely that mental health is more related to well-being than physical health per se.

3.1.1 Contemporary Concerns About Well-Being and the Reductionist Paradigm

As about the concept of health and health care, so it is about the understanding of well-being and its enhancement strategies. The recent movement of positive psychology, in its focus on studying positive subjective experiences and positive traits, which include character strengths and virtues (Seligman and Ciszksenthmihalyi 2000), seems to be *mind centred*. Even here researchers are primarily guided by the reductionist paradigm and tend to operate within the physicalistic view of the universe. For example, researchers have examined the effect of laughter on health and well-being, but most of them focus on the brain mechanisms involved and neurochemicals released rather than on the psychological aspects. No one bothers about the social aspects of it, let alone the spiritual. It is the same approach in understanding the effects of meditation or prayer, which are basically spiritual practices.

Thus, health psychology and positive psychology betray the underlying dichotomy of mind-matter dualism. Though there has been much talk of mind-body interaction in various ways and many researchers have spoken about holistic approach to health often the discussion centres on how the psychological and social, nay even spiritual aspects ultimately enhance certain neurochemicals and neurotransmitters essential for healthy functioning of the body rather than on directly addressing them.

3.1.2 Paradigm Shift: Has That Really Occurred?

What if body in itself is not all that important in maintaining health? What if mind plays a crucial role in causing illness and also in improving health? What if interpersonal and social factors also have a say in our health? What if money has no value for well-being, beyond a certain point? What if health and well-being are not always related? What if subjective criteria are more important than objective criteria for well-being? What happens to health-care industry? How do policymakers go about improving the well-being of people in a nation? What is the role of social and behavioural scientists? These and many other questions have been debated by researchers. These debates call for a paradigm shift from a purely biomedical model to a bio-psychosocial or to a holistic model that subsumes even the spiritual dimension.

Ever since Hans Selye's (1955) concept of 'general adaptation syndrome' (GAS) gained currency leading to research on life stress and strategies of coping, there has been a talk of paradigm shift in the field of medicine. Researchers focused more on psychological and social factors determining illness and recovery and also the way people manage their stress. Since then, there has been talk of 'mind-body medicine', 'psychoneuroimmunology', 'energy medicine', 'alternative medicine', 'complementary medicine', 'holistic health', 'integrative medicine', 'mind-body therapy', 'energetic therapies', 'eastern therapies' and so on (Eden 2008; Keegan 2002).

The primacy of body and body-centred approach was apparently giving way gradually to the new 'bio-psychosocial-spiritual model', which addresses the issue of illness and health taking into account not only biological functioning but also the psychological condition, social aspects and the religio-spiritual dimensions of human existence. The US National Institute of Health opened a new establishment to fund research in alternative and complementary medicine more than a decade ago. In India, a new initiative was mooted to bring together the different indigenous systems of healing under the banner AYUSH (Āyurveda, Yoga, Unani, Siddha and Homeopathy). It is interesting that this acronym also stands for life and longevity, because in Sanskrit *ayushya* means longevity. With these developments, has the paradigm shift really occurred in the world at large? Answer is no. Not much change is visible in the medical establishment all over the world, and the health industry (illness industry?) continues to thrive. Reason for this is not too difficult to find.

First, a large majority of physicians, psychiatrists, psychologists and other health professionals primarily operate within the established canons of scientific tradition. The most important of them is the fundamental assumption of primacy of materiality of the universe and hence everything has to be demonstrated at a physical level, i.e. in terms of biochemical and neurochemical activities, reactions and outcomes to be accepted as efficacious. Ajaya (1983) termed this as 'reductionist paradigm'. The fundamental assumption of this paradigm is that the only principle in the universe is matter and all other complex or abstract phenomena – be they psychological, sociological or spiritual – can be ultimately understood through a process of reduction to basic components of matter. This demand is hard to meet. Many of the so-called alternative or complementary systems involve interventions at psychological, social and even spiritual dimensions whose role in treatment outcome cannot be accounted for scientifically in the same way as it can be done with the administration of drugs. This is all the more evident when religious and spiritual aspects are part of such intervention strategies. Many researchers have tried to examine the role of spirituality in terms of prayer, healing through touch, meditation and many other means. All of them indicate that somehow our health is significantly determined by the spiritual aspect, though exact mechanisms are not understood. While there are many first person accounts of healing narrated by those who experienced it and there are a few physicians who vouch for it by and large, there is a lot of scepticism about such possibilities.

Second, there is a financial angle to this. Insurance companies pay for those treatment methods which are proven to be effective scientifically through randomized controlled trials, and there has been a greater emphasis on evidence-based practice. Consequently, investors are not willing to take risk in something not proved, lest they incur loss.

Third, there are many instances where people have not benefitted from such interventions, which further increase the scepticism towards them.

Fourth, an alternative system is chosen as second best either because the allopathic system did not work, or because they found it less expensive, or for some other reason, but not because it is more efficacious. Those who believe in the efficacy of alternative systems are few compared to the vast majority. Here again our beliefs, values and worldview seem to play a significant role.

The approach of 'one size fits all' in understanding the issues related to a disease, in the practice of intervention, in prevention of disease, in promotion of health and in the study of well-being is neither appropriate nor effective. Nor are we doing justice to the intended purposes of many of the interventions developed from an alternative perspective. In other words, however much modern psychology tries to incorporate a broader perspective on human condition, its adherence to the reductionist paradigm retards its thinking and the prospect of achieving a truly holistic perspective. So, we need to look elsewhere for an alternative way of approaching reality to overcome this drag or inertial force (*tamas* according to Indian view) of reductionism.

In this changing context, Indian perspectives on the nature of reality, on mind-body relationship and on the nature of consciousness have been found to be of much value as resources for developing the new paradigm. This chapter focuses on some of the essential elements of Indian perspectives, which are relevant and significant in this endeavour.

3.2 Perspectives on Reality in Indian Traditions

As indicated already, modern scientific approach to health and well-being as reflected in different related branches of knowledge such as medicine, psychiatry, psychology, economics and sociology is governed by the reductionist paradigm. To be more specific, it is governed by a materialist-monist view of reality, where primacy of matter is upheld. Even the Cartesian dualism of body-mind gets reduced to physical matter. Within this paradigm, mind and consciousness are viewed as synonymous, and consciousness is not accepted as an independent principle, in addition to matter. Therefore, all the issues of health and well-being are understood and dealt with materially. Even if one prays to God for better health, God is also conceptualized as a psychological resource, and the effects have to be measured in terms of the activity of the brain (neurochemistry) or of other bodily systems (biochemistry).

While such an approach may help in certain ways, it fails to take into account a macro perspective on the interrelation of different dimensions of the universe and the interplay of many factors in a grid. Though, of late, ecologists have been trying to impress upon policymakers the adverse impact on health of the human created ecological imbalance, all those arguments are again presented within the materialist-monist view of reality. There is no scope or role of any other factor. This is quite understandable given the fact that modern science started as natural philosophy in ancient Greece, which meant trying to understand the universal phenomena in naturalistic terms without invoking any supernatural principle or factor (Leahey 2004).

This view still rules the roost, despite contradictory evidences that point towards the existence of the spiritual realms beyond the perceived physical reality (Church 2007; Krippner and Friedman 2010a, b; Schwartz 2007, 2011).

In contrast to this scenario of the modern Western intellectual tradition, Indian traditions have all along affirmed the existence of multiple realities (*loka*) in the universe and a spiritual dimension to human nature that enables them to make contact with those realities. Consequently, the entire human existence is viewed with reference to a radically different perspective that may be characterized as *transcendental or spiritual* vis-à-vis the material perspective of the modern Western intellectual tradition. As a corollary, even the issues related to health and well-being are appreciated in a different way. To understand this difference, we need to elaborate on how such a perspective provides alternative views on the nature of reality and on human nature.

Indian thinkers espoused different views on reality, and we have a complete spectrum of them (Hiriyanna 1993), ranging from the absolute materialism or physicalism epitomized by Chārvaka to the dualism of Sāmkhya on to the non-dualism of Advaita Vedānta. It is important to note that there is an experiential base for such views and they are not just matters of intellectual debate or argument. Such a base can be found in the discussions on the nature of reality, self, consciousness and mind in several Upanishad and later in the Yogavāsiṣta, Bhagavad Gita and Yoga Sutras of Patanjali, just to speak of ancient original sources of sanātana dharma.

Frawley (1995) translated *sanātana dharma* as 'the eternal tradition' which literally means the 'eternal or universal truth' and is 'sometimes translated as the 'perennial wisdom' … a tradition conceived as inherent in the cosmic mind, arising with creation itself … [it] is a set of teachings which comprehend Universal Life and Consciousness, including religion, yoga and mysticism, philosophy, science, art and culture as part of a single reality' (p. 18). Frawley identified the following characteristics of *sanātana dharma*: (a) It is not limited to any messiah, prophet, scripture or church. (b) It is not restricted to any particular community or looking towards any particular historical end. (c) It embraces all aspiration towards the Divine or Supreme Being by all creatures, not only human beings but also plants and animals and the creatures, godly or ungodly, of subtle worlds beyond our physical senses. (d) It maintains our connection with the universal tradition through all worlds and all time, to the ancient past and the distant future 'in the vision of a timeless self-renewing reality (Brahman)' (1995, pp. 20–21).

We find similar ideas though not the same, in the ancient sources of Jain and Buddha traditions as well. From these, we can infer a set of fundamental assumptions, principles and practices that represent the Indian paradigm.

3.2.1 Non-dualism in Veda and Upanishad

Indian traditions subordinate physical reality to a higher spiritual reality. This is true no matter which *darsana* (perspective) it is, be it *Vedic* (Pūrva Mīmāmsa and Uttara

Mīmāmsa/Vedānta), *Vedic related* (Sāmkhya-Yoga and Nyāya-Vaisheshika) or *non-Vedic* (Jainism and Buddhism). The differences in these perspectives emerge in view of how the higher spiritual reality is conceptualized. That in turn can be speculated to arise from the nature and extent of the awareness (experiences) of the ancient seer and sages who formulated them, just as we have Freudian and Jungian psychologies. While this is not the place to review all these different perspectives, at least highlighting some of their distinctive features can be useful.

The first view is that there is only the reality that governs everything, which is designated as Brahman, and everything is its manifestation. So, there is no real duality. The apparent duality of subject-object is 'dream like', and the manifested multiplicity and variety of the world do not have substantiality. It can be compared to the holographic images projected in the sky. This view has emerged from the realization of many seers and sages of Vedic tradition, who vouch from their experience that behind and beyond the three states, viz. waking, dream and sleep, there is a fourth (*turīya*) state (Māndukya Upanishad, 12th verse) (Nikhilananda 2000). It is claimed to be pure awareness, or the awareness of awareness of the contents of mind that supports, as the ground for the figure in Gestaltian sense. It is variously termed as *sat-chit-ānanda, shuddha chaitanya, sākshi chaitanya, Purusha, Ātman* and so on in different *darsanas*.

The fact that there have been annual conferences on non-duality and science taking place for the last few years in California (SAND conferences – www.scienceandnonduality.com) and that their logo is Om = mc^2 highlights that Indian perspectives are not to be misclassified as primitive as some anthropologists of structuralist tradition attempted to do. Ken Wilber, a well-known transpersonal theorist, distinguished between the 'pre-personal' and the 'transpersonal' and pointed out that many researchers often confound the two (Wilber 1977).

Even Gautama the Buddha, who did not accept the Vedic teachings as authority and also disagreed with the notion of a permanent or eternal Self-sense (*Ātman*), did not deny a transcendental dimension of human consciousness. Some schools of Buddhist tradition also hold a non-dualistic view of reality.

3.2.2 Dualism of Sāmkhya

A second major perspective in Indian traditions posits that there are two fundamental realities instead of one. This is the perspective of *Sāmkhya* system. According to this system, both the pure consciousness and the phenomenal universe are recognized as independent realities. While the former is called *Purusha*, the latter is called *Prakṛti*. Prakṛti again is understood to be constituted of three operational principles *guṇa*, viz. *satva, rajas* and *tamas*. Each and every phenomenon in the universe – mental or material – is understood in terms of these three principles. *Sāmkhya* system derives from these two fundamental/primary realities 24 secondary principles (*tattva*) that help to account for the origin, evolution and manifestation of universal phenomena. Yoga philosophy of Patanjali is rooted in the *Sāmkhya* perspective.

The dualism of *Sāmkhya* system is different from the Cartesian dualism of mind and matter because in *Sāmkhya*, both matter and mind are viewed as the products of *satva, rajas* and *tamas* (i.e. *Prakṛti*), and hence there is no essential difference between the two. They may be considered to be on a continuum (these topics are extensively developed also in Chaps. 4, 8, 9 and 10 of this volume). Though all the three are present in what we recognize as mind and matter, gross matter is understood to be preponderant of *tamas*, while mind is understood to be preponderantly characterized by *satva* (Murthy and Kumar 2007). Though the three are described to have many characteristics, *prakāsha* (illumination, brightness) for *satva, pravrtti* (being active, being engaged) for *rajas* and *moha* (delusion, confusion) for *tamas* are regarded as the cardinal features in the Bhagavad Gita (Chapter, 14, v.22).

In the Bhagavad Gita, this dualism is described as *kshetra* and *kshetrajna* (the entire Chapter 13 is devoted to a detailed discussion of this distinction). The former is the field, and the latter is the Knower of the field. The Knower here is the absolute principle of reality, not the cognisor/subject/ego of modern psychology. For this Knower, everything else is the field that includes mind-matter continuum. For a psychological interpretation of the Bhagavad Gita, one can refer to Rama (1996).

3.2.3 Other Indian Perspectives

Jainism and Buddhism are two other major perspectives in India. Jaina tradition is believed to be as old as Vedic tradition. There seem to be a lot of mutual influence between these two traditions. Jainism has also influenced Buddhism to quite an extent.

Jainism and Buddhism, being non-Vedic in origin (meaning not accepting the authority of Vedas as revealed scriptures), do not share all the fundamental assumptions of the Vedic tradition. Yet, they also recognize the transcendental dimension of reality, the spiritual nature of humans, the notion of pure awareness, mind-matter continuum and such like.

3.3 Some Basic Assumptions and Principles Derived from Indian Perspectives

The possibility of the existence of another state beyond the three states normally experienced by all human beings relativizes the experiences of our waking state. Just as we tend to attach a secondary significance to our dream experiences, however good or bad they may be, after waking up, all the sages and saints of India have time and again asserted that even our waking state experiences lose their intensity once we 'know', i.e. experience, the higher state. The meaning and significance of pain, suffering, illness, disease, health, happiness, well-being and related constructs get radically altered.

This is not strange if we just look at it as another evolutionary possibility available to humans. What prevents us from accepting such a possibility is that it changes the figure-ground relationship to which we have accustomed to and also alters the time-space relationship, which serves as the coordinates of our daily routine. Adherence to the modern scientific framework adds to the disbelief in such a possibility, while many individuals irrespective of caste, creed, class, religion, gender, age and nationality report such experiences all over the world. Modern evolutionary perspective, with the view that humans are at the peak of evolutionary ladder, also blinds our vision to the possibility of future evolution of mankind to a higher level.

The fact that Indian thinkers recognized the evolution of man, but did not limit themselves by considering humans as the ultimate primates, enabled them to move ahead and realize other human potentialities available (see Chap. 4 for further discussions on this topic). Even the evolutionary perspective is regarded as a tale told to a child to lull it into sleep, because it has validity only from a waking standpoint. Just as a baby conceived, given birth, which grows into adulthood, marries, begets children, reaches old age and dies – all in the dream – has no reality in waking state, even the story of evolution is not valid from the ground state of consciousness.

This radical view of things is not limited to Indian seers and sages. Even mystics of other traditions in other part of the world have reiterated it. So, what we consider as Indian perspective is not exclusive or limited to India and hence universal in nature. Probably, the only difference is due to some historical or environmental or cosmological circumstance. Only Divinity perhaps knows why it is so that in India we have had more seers and sages than those entire put together elsewhere in the world, just like there are more cars in America than anywhere else in the world. So our lifestyle has been determined by the vision of those ancient ones, and it continues to operate till date. We can summarize the Indian viewpoint as below.

Indian tradition upholds that (a) the spiritual reality can be perceived through intuitive faculty; (b) the soul is independent of body; (c) consciousness, *cit*, is different from mind/psyche; (d) body and mind are constituted of the same three properties or *guṇa* – *triguṇa* – and hence they are not different in substance; (e) there is life after death; (f) there are paranormal phenomena which can be experienced; and (g) a human being can attain liberation from the cycle of birth and death through Self-realization. These and other related beliefs have shaped the way of life in the Indian subcontinent leading to a holistic perspective, in which a human being is understood as biological, psychological and spiritual in nature and is in constant relation with the whole cosmos.

3.3.1 *Triguṇa*

Among the above central themes and concepts, the one that has far-reaching implications for understanding the happenings in the universe is *triguṇa*, already referred to in Sect. 3.2.2. This concept had its origins in the Vedas but was further developed in the *Sāmkhya* perspective and has been found to be useful by all other systems.

The concept of the three *guṇa* (*satva, rajas* and *tamas*) is widely used to understand the properties of gross physical matter and its various inorganic and organic manifestations in nature and also in accounting for psychological, social and religio-spiritual phenomena. Hence, this concept has attracted the attention of psychologists, and there have been many attempts to develop scales to understand the personality with reference to the three *guṇa* (Murthy and Kumar 2007).

The three *guṇa* (also discussed in Chaps. 4, 9 and 10) operate in all the persons, and the ancient literature has described the trait characteristics of those who are predominantly governed by one of them. But these are not absolute, and it is quite common that in a given situation or state, a person may be governed by a *guṇa* other than the one which chiefly characterizes that person. Hence, the operation of *guṇa* in human beings can be understood both as state and trait. Indian systems have understood illness and disease as products of the predominance and malfunctioning of *rajas* and *tamas* and health and well-being as the predominance of *satva*, both at the level of a person and at social or even cosmic level. Increase in *rajas* and *tamas* leads to negativity, and increase in *satva* leads to positivity. Since the three *guṇa* always remain everywhere, the action and reaction, cause and effect are understood with reference to them for everything. Just to take a simple example, if one consumes more chillies, which is supposed to have an energizing property, it is *rajas* that is acting and overacting to bring about certain effects. On the other hand, drinking milk has the calming effect, and it is *satva* which is acting.

Since the *triguṇa* system allows for the interaction of mind and matter, a systemic view is possible in which person and the environment mutually influence each other, wherein the predominance of one of the three *guṇa* can affect one way or another. Whether it is ecological imbalance at the macrocosmic level, biochemical imbalance at the microcosmic level or cognitive/affective/conative disturbance at psychological level, all are viewed as manifestations of negativity, and harmony at all levels is understood in terms of positivity (as highlighted in Chaps. 5 and 10 of this volume). Thus, illness or disease and health and well-being of a locale, a person, a society, a nation or a culture reflect the dynamic equilibrium of the three *guṇa*. For example, increased violence, aggression, crime, sexual assaults, corruption and such other negative behaviours across globe are manifestations of increased dominance of *rajas* and *tamas* over *satva*; so also the natural calamities and man created calamities occurring all over the world. Understanding of global events in this way has led to another popular conceptualization known as *tāpa traya*.

3.3.2 *Tāpa Traya*

The word *tāpa* means heat. It generates suffering and therefore is metaphorically equated with suffering. *Traya* is three, and suffering is of three kinds originating from three different sources, viz. physical (*bhautika*), supernatural (*daivika*) and self (*ātmika*) since reality has many dimensions. *Ādibhautika* refers to all kinds of suffering originating from physical or material causes, including environmental factors, natural calamities, accidents, other physical beings – animal and human, and all kinds of physical or material factors. *Ādidaivika* refers to all kinds of suffering originating from discarnate entities and beings. *Ādyatmika* refers to all kinds of suffering originated from personal factors – biological, psychological and social. Thus, human suffering can take any form, and disease and illness are one such manifestation.

Therefore, in Indian tradition, a person's health and well-being are understood not only with reference to gross physical body and its functional status but also in relation to one's mental status and supernatural aspects. A person's illness, disease, health and well-being may be influenced by one or more of these factors, and hence they are understood multidimensionally. Thus, a person suffering from a prolonged illness could be due to something that happened in this life in the physical world or it may have been due to the action of a supernatural factor or it could have its origin in the activities of a previous life or it could be due to one's mental factors and so on. Since the past can carry its effect into the present, present can equally affect the future. Similarly, even health and well-being are also understood with reference to past, present and future. Thus, interventions required have to be appropriate to the dimension of reality from which the suffering has originated. This is reflected in Āyurveda (which means theory and practice of longevity, not just medicine) that speaks of three kinds of intervention: *yuktivyapāshraya, daivavyapāshraya* and *sattvāvajaya,* which correspond to the three origins of suffering. The first one involves all kinds of medical treatment, also known as *kāya chikitsa* (treatment for the body); the second refers to all kinds of practices that are aimed at influencing supernatural forces, also known as *bhoota vidya*; and the third refers to psychological therapy and counselling which involves restrengthening *sātvic* tendency.

It is to be noted here that the concept of *tāpa traya* is meaningful only when one understands it in the context of how a human being is viewed in Indian traditions. The recognition and affirmation of the spiritual/transcendental dimension of human nature led ancient Indian seer and sages to view human being as bi-dimensional rather than uni-dimensional. In other words, human being is not understood only in terms of gross physical body but also in terms of an extracorporeal soul/spirit that transcends the limits of the physical body as well as the notion of space and time. It is not that people and thinkers in other parts of the globe have not recognized this dimension. The distinctiveness of India in this issue is its consistent and continuous affirmation of this dimension for the past thousands of years and upholding that as the primary aspect of human nature rather than gross physical body.

This feature comes through very explicitly and forcefully in one of the verses of the Bhagavad Gita, which when translated in English reads as follows: 'just as humans throw away a torn cloth/dress and wear a new one, the one who is in this body takes upon a new one when it gets worn out (dies)' (Chap. 2 v. 22) (translation author's). This distinction between *dehi* (own who is in the body or owns the body) and *deha* (gross physical body) is fundamental in shaping the traditional views on illness, suffering, health and well-being. It has made possible for people in India to view the body as something that takes birth, develops/grows and decays and dies eventually just as a plant or an animal. That provides a detached perspective on one's body and understands illness and health, disease and recovery, treatment and cure in a more natural way.

This distinction has also shaped the way such events as death are expressed linguistically, with reference to *dehi* rather than *deha.* For example, in Kannada language, which is my mother tongue, it is said *jīva hoitu* (soul has gone). Since *dehi* or *jīva* is the same as *prāna*, life force, *prāna hoitu* (life force has gone) is also another usage to refer to death. In Sanskrit literature and its derivatives, the *prāna* is also equated with a bird, *pakshi*, and one's death is referred to metaphorically as the flying away of a bird from its nest. One can find such expressions in all the Indian languages.

There are two important aspects here which require further elaboration. First, since the gross physical body is not viewed as the primary aspect of a human being, it does not get more attention than what it is due, either in birth or death or during one's life. Compared to Western culture, where lifestyle predominantly centres on primary bodily needs and its secondary elaborations, Indian culture is centred on *dehi* or *jīva*, its terrestrial and transmigratory existence and the eventual release from the cycle of birth and death. Therefore, it is the culture of the soul that is practised rather than culture of the body. Sixteen culturing rites and rituals (*shodasha samskāra*) are practised, starting from the stage of conception to death, aimed at the development of the soul first, and only secondarily of the body, for it is the soul which is on its journey from one bodily existence to the other (the importance of rituals for health and well-being is thoroughly discussed in Chap. 6). Soul in this journey can continue to actualize its immense potential for which body is a vehicle. Thus, a yogi can leave his/her body and enter a dead body (*para kāya pravesha*), dismantle one's limbs and torso and reassemble (*khanda yoga*), cast of his/her aged or worn out body at will (*prāyopavesha*), manifest simultaneously in more than one place, transfer one's youthfulness to an aged person, take on someone else's physical illness and consciously suffer, self-cure one's dreaded diseases and what not.

While the above examples are exceptions rather than rule and only adept yogi could do all that, they are cited here to illustrate the fact that ancient Indian seer and sages were well aware of the immense hidden potentialities of the soul that can manifest through the body and hence cared and protected their body as an instrument rather than body as the only living reality. Towards this end, they had developed very sophisticated understanding of bodily organs and functions and their maintenance, which modern medical science is yet to come to terms with.

There is enough traditional knowledge and wisdom available in folklore as well as in classical texts related to medicine about how to care for the body from birth to death. What it means is life of a human being was/is not construed in terms of bodily existence alone, thereby attaching all the importance to bodily security and bodily needs. In other words, it was/is not body centred still, despite all the modern innovations like ventilators, pacemakers, plastic surgeries, transplantation and implantations. The idea that body is like a cloth that gets worn out in due course is an integral part of the Indian psyche.

If this is so, then how do we understand the place of body in human existence; what is the purpose of bodily existence; what is the relation of body, mind and soul;

and what is the meaning of illness, disease, suffering, death, health, well-being and so on? All the Indian systems have dealt with these issues as their central concern. Gautama the prince became Buddha the realized one, in course of finding answer to these questions. It is not possible to review all the different answers found by ancient seer and sages for these questions. But what can be discussed is how their insights shaped the cultural outlook of Indian civilization in general and issues related to health and well-being in particular.

3.3.3 Perspectives on the Constitution of Human Beings

Though we speak so much about psychology and psychological effects, the existence of mind, soul and Self remains controversial. However, in Indian traditions, soma (body), psyche (soul/mind) and spirit (Self) are recognized as aspects of a human being, and their experiential validity is affirmed time and again. In other words, man is regarded as a complex of biological, psychological and spiritual features.

In *Kathopanishad* (a.k.a Kāthakopanishad), there is the metaphor of a chariot, *ratha*, which describes the relationship between these three as follows: 'one has to understand the 'self' as the person seated in a chariot and the 'body' as the chariot; '*buddhi*' has to be considered as the charioteer; '*manas*' as the bridle and the 'sense-organs' as horses' (I, 3, 3–4) (Hiriyanna 2004). As Jadunath Sinha (1961) has noted, in this framework of understanding, *manas* is superior to sense organs; *buddhi*, intellect, is superior to *manas*; self is superior to *buddhi*; and there is nothing superior to the Self. The self mentioned here is identified with the supreme Self (Brahman). From the Upanishadic point of view, the mind-body complex is an organ of experience subordinated to the Self. The body, sense organs, *manas* and *buddhi* exist for the Self, but the Self exists for itself, and there is no reality beyond it (Sinha 1961). It is spiritual in nature and is different from the bio-psychosocial identity or self-senses that we develop in our lifetime, which leads to a conditional existence.

In *Taittiriya Upanishad*, the same idea is expressed in a different way, with another metaphor: *kosha*. In this Upanishad (Section 2 – Ānandavalli), spiritual Self is characterized as *ānandamaya* and is distinguished from the other four *koshas* ordinarily translated as sheaths. They are labelled *annamaya* (gross physical body), *prānamaya* (vital or life force), *manomaya* (emotions and drives) and *vijnānamaya* (discriminative intellect and intuitive functions). From *Taittiriya Upanishad* point of view, a person's innermost essence or Self is itself blissful, *ānandamaya*, and at the core all human beings have unbounded joy. However, people do not realize this because this inner core is covered by the four sheaths from subtlest (*vijnānamaya*) to grossest (*annamaya*).

A third way of understanding human being that we come across in Indian tradition is in terms of three types of body, viz. *sthūla sharīra, sōkshma sharīra* and *kārana sharīra*. *Sthūla sharīra* refers to gross physical body. *Sōkshma sharīra* also called *linga sharīra* termed as subtle body is understood as constituted of *prānamaya*, *manomaya* and *vijnānamaya kosha* as described in *Taittiriya Upanishad*. *Kārana sharīra*, termed as causal body, represents the *ānandamaya* of *Taittiriya Upanishad*, and deep sleep is the manifestation of causal body (Chap. 5 further describes the three bodies). Beyond these three bodies is the *Ātman*, which is self-luminous, pure, immutable and eternally free – the witness of the three empirical conditions of waking, dream and deep sleep, and different from the five sheaths (Sinha 1961).

Hence, according to Indian traditions, when one realizes spiritual nature, his/her locus of identity shifts from biological and psychosocial aspects to newly found spiritual nature, and the person attains an inner sense of 'peace', 'tranquillity' and 'bliss', even if one is having some problem at the levels of the gross and subtle body. Therefore, Indian traditions hold that the ultimate sense of well-being is not contingent upon the absence of physical or psychological ailment. We have in India plenty of instances of *mahātma* (as in Mahātma Gandhi, meaning an evolved soul) and *jeevanmukta* (a person who is liberated from the cycle of birth and death through Self-realization) who did suffer from certain physical diseases and yet could remain in a state of bliss like Sri Ramana Maharshi who underwent surgical intervention for a malignant cancerous growth without anaesthesia three times (see Swamy 1985).

Thus, from traditional Indian point of view, all issues related to disease, illness, therapy and treatment are applicable only to gross physical body (*sthūla sharīra*) and to what is understood as subtle body (*sōkshma sharīra*), *not* to *Ātman*, which is free from all kinds of afflictions. Thus, health and well-being defined with reference to gross and subtle bodies are considered relative, and one is urged to attain the supreme well-being, which is associated with *Atma sākshātkāra*, Self-realization.

If we really think about the Cartesian differentiation of *res cogitans* and *res extensa*, and also his famous statement *cogito ergo sum* (I think, therefore I am), we find that Descartes was very near to Indian thought, except that he located himself or his identity at the thinking principle, whereas Indian seer and sages went beyond that and affirmed another level of identity, viz. *I am, therefore I am*.

While all the Indian systems recognized that level as pure awareness, different systems spoke of it in different ways.[2] Veda, Upanishads and other Vedic related systems called this level as *Ātman*, the *Sāmkhya* referred to it as *Purusha*, Bhagavad Gita called it *kshetrajna* and Patanjali in his Yoga Sutra called it *drashtu*. But Buddha refrained from equating it with any first-person references. Whatever may be the difference, the fact remains that the Indian systems recognized a level of *ground awareness*. It is interesting, as I type this chapter sitting here in Conway, I remember the difference in how we refer to the different floors of a building. What we refer to as ground floor in India is termed as first floor in the USA. But the site of demolished World Trade Centre is referred to as Ground Zero, because there are no buildings and floors any more. What Indian thinkers are referring to is such a *Ground Zero State of Consciousness*.

Operationally, this state has two aspects: intelligence/awareness/consciousness and energy. The term *caitanya* embodies both of these connotations. So to have

[2] *Ekam sat viprā bahudā vadanti – Truth is one but knowledgeable persons speak of it differently (trans. author's).*

realization of this fundamental principle is to be omniscient, omnipresent and omnipotent. This can only be realized when one wakes up from a 'grand dream'.

The seers and sages who had this realization (a) could manipulate the forces of nature at will, (b) could be present simultaneously at different dimensions, (c) could affect changes at distance and (d) could intervene in the life of people for their good from a cosmic perspective and remove their *karma*. They were also embodiment of great compassion, love, altruism, wisdom and such other virtues. They were the real *Guru*, not the contemporary corrupt usage of that term appended to all kinds of persons whether they have really attained that level or not.

In the presence of such great Guru, healing happens, illness gets cured, health improves and the ultimate sense of well-being termed as *ānanda* is attained. All this happens whether a person is near or far physically, because the 'presence of a Guru' is not the bodily presence, it is the presence of a spiritual kind. Autobiographies and biographies of many great masters, day-to-day recordings in the presence of such masters and first-person accounts of people who underwent healing experiences shared in print in popular and academic sources document the myriad instances of suffering being removed.

This sounds like a fairy tale to many, but there have been records and testimonies of the existence of many such personages who include modern mystics and sages of the twentieth century.

3.4 Implications for Health and Well-Being Research and Practice

In the recent past, more and more researchers are willing to believe in mind and its effects, though their views on mind differ. While some accept it as independent of body, others consider it as an emergent phenomenon of the activity of the brain. Either way it has been possible for researchers to speak of psychophysiological disorders, mind-body medicine, psychosomatic medicine, and psychoneuroimmunology, all resulting in bio-psychosocial models of illness and health. However, beliefs in a soul and Self are a far cry, and holistic approaches which incorporate all the three aspects of human nature are rare.

More recently, a new field known as 'energy psychology' has emerged, which essentially deals with notions that are similar to the concepts of *sōkshma sharīra* and *kārana sharīra*. Though we in India do not have scientific research to prove the existence of *sōkshma sharīra* and *kārana sharīra* as described in our tradition, some of the research studies conducted in Western countries on energy fields or aura around the human body (referred to as subtle body) using imaging techniques such as Kirlian photography lend some support to such a conceptualization. Such researches and personal experiences of people there have led many Westerners to take the concept of *chakra* seriously

Chakra is a Sanskrit term, which literally means a 'wheel'. In the present context, it refers to centres of energy located across the human spine, from lumbar region to the vortex/top of the head. They are totally seven in number. As Dale (2011) puts it, 'chakras regulate, maintain, and manage the physical, emotional, mental, and spiritual aspects of our being on the physical plane. Chakras themselves serve as revolving doors or portals between our body, mind, and soul' (p. 23). The reports of people who are endowed with clairvoyant abilities have provided some additional evidence confirming the conceptualization of subtle and causal body (Dale 2009, 2011; Lockhart 2010).

Further, recent popularization of healing practices such as 'pranic healing' and 'reiki', which are known to operate on energy fields around gross physical body, may be treated as another indirect evidence for the existence of subtle and causal dimensions of human nature (Eden 2008). Many of the traditional healing practices prevalent in India operate at these levels. Similarly, research on 'out-of-body experiences' (OBEs), 'near-death experiences' (NDEs) and 'reincarnation' cases conducted by both Western and Indian researchers (Krippner, and Friedman 2010a, b) may also be taken as possible supportive evidence for the Indian belief system.

Second, in Indian traditional society, metaphysical beliefs – in *karma*, in God's will and in spirits – are presumed to be important determinants of many events in one's life including diseases and suffering of all kinds. *Karma* or *karmaphala* refers to the suffering that is frequently attributed to one's own misdeeds in this and/or previous lives. God's will refers to the control of an external agent or power that governs reward and punishment, not always according to what one deserves. Fate implies that all life events are predestined and one can do little to alter them (Kohli and Dalal 1998). Hence, Indian tradition holds that disease and illness can be understood as one manifestation of human suffering. A more recent development in the Western world that lends some theoretical and empirical evidence is what is known as *information medicine* (McTaggart 2008a, b; http://www.thelivingmatrixmovie.com).

These developments are interpreted with reference to the quantum view of the universe, which is again coming closer to the non-dual and dualistic view of reality espoused in the Indian traditions (in Chap. 8 the parallelism between quantum logic and Vedic view of the universe is deeply discussed). While the dualist view of two fundamental realities of *purusha* and *prakṛti* can be used as a framework to understand, many healing approaches that involve invoking a higher power, the spontaneous healing that take place in the presence of mystics or in sacred places could be explained with reference non-dual perspective.

While the positive psychology movement is hotly debating on the nature and sources of happiness and well-being, the ancient Indian seer and sage went a step ahead and declared that the fundamental or essential sense of well-being lies in the transcendental dimension and characterized it as *ānanda*. They did not make any distinction in the quality of happiness associated with the material life and the spiritual life. On the other hand, they treated *ānanda* as the basic experience and regarded happiness related to mundane life as an aspect of this essential experience. They also spoke of well-being as *preyas* and *shreyas*, the former corresponding to the material and social levels of reality and the latter to the transcendental level of reality. Contemporary distinction between hedonic and eudaimonic happiness corresponds to *preyas*. Ancient seer and sages as well as modern ones have along pointed out that *shreyas* is what matters ultimately (Salagame 2012).

3.5 Modes of Intervention from the Indian Perspective

In view of the multidimensional outlook on human nature and his/her suffering, the modes of therapy and treatment range from the most mundane to the highly spiritual, according to the level at which disease and illness are understood to have occurred. To put it in medical terminology, the relation of symptomatology to aetiology and pathology is governed by ontology, and therefore the modes of intervention become multimodal.

Anand et al. (2001) have noted that healing systems differ in terms of explanations of suffering, healing techniques and the types of healers. They distinguish between three types of healers: (a) Professional healers, known as *vaid* (*vaidya*) and *hakim*, who deal primarily with physical suffering though they frequently practice what we can call 'psychological medicine'. This corresponds to physical/bodily origin of problems (*ādhyatmika*) already referred to in Sect. 3.3.2. (b) Folk and popular healers, who include palmists, horoscope specialists, herbalists, diviners, sorcerers (a variety of shamans) and *ojhas*. Their healing techniques draw from astrology, medicine, alchemy and magic and thrive on folk and popular beliefs and practices. (c) Mystical-spiritual healers, who include *sādhus*, saints, priests, and *swāmis*. They primarily work on the religious faiths and belief systems of the community. While a vaidya or hakim may address problems related to *ādhyatmika* source, the other two – folk and mystic-spiritual healers – address problems emerging from all the three *ādibhautika, ādidaivika* and *ādhyatmika* sources According to these researchers, all these traditional healing practices share an element of mysticism and a flavour of sacredness; they thrive on myths, legends, history, rituals and belief systems of the local communities; and cultural symbolism is used to bring about a transformation of consciousness (see Chaps. 6 and 7 in relation to these topics).

Thus, it is to be noted that Indian perspectives on health and well-being gain a wider meaning than how it is understood in modern medicine, psychiatry and psychology. Health and well-being of a person are integral aspect of the health and well-being of the cosmos as a whole. Hence, the prayers – *lokāh samasthāh sukhinobhavantu* – let the whole cosmos be well or let everyone in all the worlds be well; *sarve santu sukhinah, sarve santu nirāmaya, sarve bhadrāni pashyantu, ma kashid dukhabhagbhavet, Om Shānti, Shānti, Shānti* – let everyone be well, let everyone remain at ease, let everyone have an auspicious view or outlook, let not sorrow afflict any one, Om peace, peace, peace (author's translation).

References

Ajaya, S. (1983). *Psychotherapy east and west: A unifying paradigm*. Honesdale: Himalayan International Institute for Yoga Sciences.

Anand, J., Srivastava, A., & Dalal, A. K. (2001). Where suffering ends and healing begins. *Psychological Studies, 48*(3), 114–126.

Brief, A. P., Butcher, A. H., George, J. M., & Link, K. E. (1993). Integrating bottom-up and top-down theories of subjective well-being: The case of health. *Journal of Personality and Social Psychology, 64*(4), 646–653.

Church, D. (2007). *The genie in your genes: Epigenetic medicine and the new biology of intention*. Santa Rosa: Elite books.

Conceição, P., & Bandura, R. (2013). *Measuring subjective wellbeing: A summary review of the literature*. http://www.undp.org/developmentstudies/docs/subjective_wellbeing_conceicao_bandura.pdf

Dale, C. (2009). *The subtle body: An encyclopedia of your energetic anatomy*. Boulder: Sounds True.

Dale, C. (2011). *The complete book of chakra healing*. Woodbury: Llewellyn Publications.

Diener, E. (1984). Subjective well-being. *Psychological Bulletin, 95*, 542–575.

Diener, E., & Seligman, M. E. P. (2004). Beyond money: Toward an economy of well-being. *Psychological Science in the Public Interest, 5*, 1–31.

Dimatteo, M. R., & Martin, L. R. (2007). *Health psychology*. New Delhi: Pearson Education.

Eden, D. (2008). *Energy medicine: Balancing your body's energies for optimal health, joy and vitality*. New York: Jeremy P. Tarcher/Penguin.

Frawley, D. (1995). *Hinduism – The eternal tradition (Sanātana Dharma)*. New Delhi: Voice of India.

Hiriyanna, M. (1993). *Outlines of Indian philosophy*. Delhi: Motilal Banarsidass Publishers Pvt. Ltd.

Hiriyanna, M. (2004). *Kāthakōpanishad with the commentary of Sri Sankarāchārya*. (Translated into English). Mysore: Kavyalaya Publishers.

Hoorn, A. (2007, April 2–3). *Is happiness measurable and what do those measures mean for policy?* International Conference. Organised by the Bank of Italy, the Centre for Economic & International Studies (CEIS), the Joint Research Centre of the European Commission and the Organisation for Economic Cooperation and Development (OECD), University of Rome 'Tor Vergata'.

Keegan, L. (2002). *Healing with complementary and alternative therapies*. Singapore: Thomson Asia Pvt. Ltd.

Kohli, N., & Dalal, A. K. (1998). Culture as a factor in causal understanding of illness: A study of cancer patients. *Psychology and Developing Societies, 10*(2), 115–129.

Krippner, S., & Friedman, H. L. (Eds.). (2010a). *Debating psychic experience: Human potential or human illusion*. Santa Barbara: Praeger.

Krippner, S., & Friedman, H. L. (Eds.). (2010b). *Mysterious minds: The neurobiology of psychics, mediums and other extraordinary people*. Santa Barbara: Praeger.

Leahey, T. H. (2004). *A history of psychology: Main currents in psychological thought* (6th ed.). New Delhi: Pearson Education.

Lockhart, M. (2010). *The subtle energy body: The complete guide*. Rochester: Inner Traditions.

McTaggart, L. (2008a). *The field: The quest for the secret force of the universe*. New York: Harper Collins.

McTaggart, L. (2008b). *The intention experiment*. New York: Free Press.

Murthy, P. K., & Kumar, S. K. K. (2007). Concept *triguṇa*: A critical analysis and synthesis. *Psychological Studies, 52*, 2.

Nikhilananda, S. (2000). *The Māndūkya Upanishad with Gaudapāda karaka and Shankar's commentary* (Translated from Sanskrit). Calcutta: Advaita Ashrama.

Rama, S. (1996). *Perennial psychology of the Bhagavad Gita*. Honesdale: The Himalayan Institute of Yoga Science and Philosophy of the U.S.A.

Salagame, K. K. K. (2012). Chapter 28: Well-being from the perspective of Hindu/Sanātana dharma. In S. David, I. Boniwal, & A. C. Ayers (Eds.), *The Oxford handbook of happiness*. Oxford: The Oxford University Press.
Schwartz, G. E. (2007). *The energy healing experiments: Science reveals our natural powers to heal*. New York: Atria Books.
Schwartz, G. E. (2011). *The sacred promise: How science is discovering spirit's collaboration with us in our daily lives*. New York: Atria Books.
Seligman, M. E., & Ciszksenthmihalyi, M. (2000). Positive psychology: An introduction. *American Psychologist, 55*(1), 5–14.
Selye, H. (1955, October 7). Stress and disease. *Science, 122*, 625–631.
Sheldon, K. M., Kashdan, T. B., & Steger, M. F. (2011). *Designing positive psychology*. New York: Oxford University Press.
Sinha, J. (1961). *Indian psychology: Vol. 2. Emotion and will*. Delhi: Motilal Banarasidas. (Reprint 1996).
Swamy, B. V. N. (1985). *Self-realization: The life and teachings of Sri Ramana Maharshi*. Tiruvannamalai: Sri Ramanashramam.
Taittiriya Upanishad – Section 2 – Anandavalli.
Watchel, P. (1989). *The poverty of affluence – A psychological portrait of the American way of life*. New York: New Society Publishers.
Wilber, K. (1977). *The spectrum of consciousness*. Wheaton Hill: The Theosophical Publishing.

Chapter 4
Concept of Health in Āyurveda

P. Ram Manohar

4.1 Introduction

Āyurveda defines itself as the science or knowledge of life (Yadavji 1980), and its primary focus is on the quality and span of life. Classical texts define Āyurveda as that which enables the individual to obtain and know life (Suśruta Saṃhitā Sūtra Sthāna 1, 15 in Yadavji 1980).

The formal definition of Āyurveda as expounded in the *Ćaraka Saṃhitā* states that Āyurveda is the body of knowledge that describes the wholesome, unwholesome, happy and unhappy states of life as well as what is wholesome and unwholesome for life, in addition to defining the span of life (Cited in Ćaraka Saṃhitā, Sūtra Sthāna, 1, 41 in Yadavji 1992). This definition succinctly summarises the subject matter of Āyurveda and makes it clear that Āyurveda is a science of health management more than being a medical system.

In another context, the same text defines Āyurveda as the knowledge that informs about substances, properties and actions that are supportive of and antagonistic to life (Cited in Ćaraka Saṃhitā, Sūtra Sthāna, 30, 23 in Yadavji 1992).

The primary goal of Āyurveda is therefore preservation of life. Longevity is the ultimate endpoint of Ayurvedic interventions. However, longevity has no meaning if it is not accompanied by health and well-being. The parameters for determining quality of life are, therefore, based on the tripod of life, health and wellness in Āyurveda (Harisastri 2002). By adopting the healthy lifestyle outlined here, one attains longevity, health and prosperity at the same time (Aṣṭāṅga Hṛdaya Saṃhitā, Sūtra Sthāna, 2, 48 in Harisastri 2002)

Āyurveda distinguishes between timely and untimely death and explains that medical science has meaning and relevance in human life because premature death can be prevented (Sharma 2012). There are hundred types of untimely death

P.R. Manohar (✉)
AVP Research Foundation, Coimbatore, Tamil Nadu, India
e-mail: rammanoharp@gmail.com

A. Morandi and A.N. Narayanan Nambi (eds.), *An Integrated View of Health and Well-being*, Cross-Cultural Advancements in Positive Psychology 5, DOI 10.1007/978-94-007-6689-1_4,

and only one timely death (Aṣṭāṅga Saṃgraha, Sūtra Sthāna 9, 89 in Sharma 2012). The latter is like the wearing out of a chariot that happens naturally in course of time, and untimely death is like the premature damage to a chariot that happens due to rough use (Aṣṭāṅga Saṃgraha, Sūtra Sthāna, 9, 95 in Sharma 2012).

To find out the ways and means to live the full human life span has been the primary goal of Āyurveda. For this reason, Āyurveda characterises itself as the knowledge of life (*Āyus* (life), *Veda* (knowledge)) rather than as a medical system. The opening chapters of the classical canon of medicine, the *Ćaraka Saṃhitā*, are therefore named as the quest for longevity (*dīrghaṃjīvitīyam*) (Yadavji 1992). Sage Bharadvāja set out to the abode of the King of Gods, Indra, to obtain the knowledge that will give a long life (Ćaraka Saṃhitā, Sūtra Sthāna, 1, 3 in Yadavji 1992).

Vedic literature is replete with prayers for living the full life span. One mantra goes thus: 'May we live a hundred autumns, may we witness a hundred autumns' (Sahebrao 2009). Another mantra aspires that the ears hear and the eyes see what is auspicious and that we live the full life span with healthy organs (Sahebrao 2009). The classical texts of Āyurveda reaffirm these sentiments stating that the human life span is a hundred years and that by adopting a healthy lifestyle, it is possible to live the full potential.

It is interesting to note that these prayers aim for collective well-being, hinting at the importance of collective human effort and participation to create the social and environmental conditions conducive for healthy life span (see Chap. 3 for further discussion of this topic). The *Ćaraka Saṃhitā* makes a distinction between wholesome, unwholesome, happy and unhappy states of life reconciling the conflict between personal and communal well-being. Public health and the wellness of the community as a whole has been given importance in Āyurveda. In accordance with the tenets of the *Sāṃkhya* system of thought, Āyurveda posits that there are three stressors in human life that lead to mental and physical illness and suffering. These emanate from within the individual (*adhyātma*), from the external environment (*ādhibhautika*) and by the act of providence (*ādhidaivika*) (Yadavji 1980).

There are three types of stressors that include the self, the environment and beyond. Therefore, sorrow in the form of disease originates from three sources—the individual, the external environment and by the act of providence (Suśruta Saṃhitā Sūtra Sthāna 24, 4–5 in Yadavji 1980).

It is from this perspective that Āyurveda evolved a community-based and ecological approach to health management. Forming the right relationships and networks between the individual and the world at large in a dynamic manner constitutes the basis of good health (see Chaps. 6 and 7 for a thorough discussion on this point).

Longevity and healthy ageing are primary twin goals of Āyurveda and come within the purview of preventive medicine. Preventive medicine is known as *Svastha Vṛtta* in Āyurveda and is not a defensive approach to maintenance of health. Āyurveda has developed a model of wellness as well as illness, and the *Ćaraka Saṃhitā* clarifies that the purpose of Āyurveda is twofold, preventive and curative (Yadavji 1992). The purpose of this treatise is twofold—the preservation of health in the healthy and cure of the sick (Ćaraka Saṃhitā, Sūtra Sthāna, 30, 26 in Yadavji 1992).

Āyurveda advocates a proactive and interventional approach to promote higher levels of health. In fact, Āyurveda emphasises that even the so-called healthy individual needs to be treated to enhance immunity and health (Yadavji 1992). Medicines or interventions are of two kinds—one that enhances the health of the healthy and the other that cures the sick (Ćaraka Saṃhitā, Cikitsā Sthāna, 1, 1–4 in Yadavji 1992).

The section on treatment of diseases in the *Ćaraka Saṃhitā* begins with chapters that deal with the enhancement of health in relatively healthy individuals (Yadavji 1992). Interestingly, the first two chapters in the section on treatments in the *Ćaraka Saṃhitā* deal with ageing and reproductive medicine. By this arrangement, it is being hinted that even a healthy individual needs to be treated systematically to enhance immunity and the quality of the tissues.

Health is considered to be an outcome of an evolutionary and adaptive process of interaction between the individual and the environment. Āyurveda defines health as the harmonious interactions with appropriate objects in the world at the appropriate moments. In other words, the right responses to relevant spatio-temporal matrices in which the individual gets embedded in the journey of life lead to healthy outcomes (a thorough discussion of this point is provided in Chap. 5). For this reason, a key determinant of health is awareness of self and environment and optimal responses to ever-changing external stimuli. Health is to be cultivated through an evolutionary process of learning by actions based on informed decisions. In the ultimate analysis, it is the lack of awareness known as *prajñāparādha* that is identified as the root cause of disease and untimely death.

To respond appropriately to situations requires awareness of self and environment. Āyurveda defines the healthy individual as *svastha*, one who is centred in the self or acts from awareness of the self when responding to the changing situations in the external environment. It is this insight that underpins the personalised or person-centred approach to medicine in Āyurveda.

Āyurveda has been propounded to discover customised solutions for the individual, known as the karma puruṣa who gropes in the spatio-temporal matrix of existence seeking life, health and longevity (Yadavji 1992). The conscious person is the focus of Āyurveda, and it is for the sake of the person that this knowledge has been propounded (Ćaraka Saṃhitā, Sūtra Sthāna, 1, 47 in Yadavji 1992). *Karma puruṣa* means the active person who is perpetually interacting with and responding to the external and internal environment. Āyurveda emphasises that a person-centred approach is indispensable because each individual is unique in terms of the mind, body, social relationships, spiritual outlook and so on and so forth.

The cornerstone of the Ayurvedic approach to personalised medicine is the concept of physical and mental constitution. Every individual is a complex and unique expression of the dynamic interaction of their physical and mental make-up. The mental constitution determines whether the individual engages in the world with awareness, emotion or ignorance. The physical constitution determines whether the biological processes are oriented towards conservation, transformation or utilisation of energy. The constitution of the individual sets certain limits as well as scope for the individual to climb the ladder of higher levels of health.

Health is a state of equilibrium, the optimal balance in the process of preservation, transformation and utilisation of energy that results in structural as well as functional integrity of the body leading to a state of comfort and ease of the senses, mind and self. *Suśruta* puts forth this idea explicitly in his famous definition of health:

> When the physiological functions, digestion and metabolism, the structural elements and the process of excretion are in balance, then one's self, sense organs and mind are at ease characterising the state of perfect health (*Suśruta Saṃhitā* Sūtra Sthāna 1, 15 in Yadavji 1980)

Āyurveda attempts to discover the optimal way to balance the body and mind with proper understanding of the constitution of the individual that will enable to establish the right relationships with the external environment.

4.2 Longevity and Healthy Ageing

Longevity is the primary goal of Āyurveda, and this goes hand in hand with healthy ageing. Āyurveda considers ageing as a disease and therefore as a condition that can be treated (Yadavji 1992):

> These interventions pacify the disease of old age and confers cognitive powers and memory (Ćaraka Saṃhitā, Cikitsa Sthāna, 3, 27 in Yadavji 1992)

The branch of Rasāyana, which improves immunity and delays ageing, is said to be a remedy for the disease of old age. It is a fundamental precept in Āyurveda that humans can not only live the full life span but also age healthily without cognitive decline and physical debility (Yadavji 1992):

> By implementing the rejuvenative treatment, one can attain long life span, memory, cognition, health as well as youthfulness. (Ćaraka Saṃhitā, Cikitsa Sthāna, 1, 7 in Yadavji 1992)

However, the foundation for healthy ageing has to be laid at a young age and not later than the middle age of an individual (Sharma 2012). There is a limit to what can be done after old age has set in:

> Rasāyana or rejuvenative therapy must be performed before ageing sets in in the early or middle phases of life (Aṣṭāṅga Hṛdaya, Uttara Sthāna, 39, 3 in Harisastri 2002)

In fact, Āyurveda has observed that interventions have to be initiated at the stage of conception itself to enhance the quality of life in late stages (Harisastri 2002). Physical constitution is formed at the time of conception and, like the genetic make-up of the individual, cannot be changed (Aṣṭāṅga Hṛdaya, Sūtra Sthāna, 1, 9–10 in Harisastri 2002). Detoxification programmes and strengthening of the tissues through structured interventions aim to enhance and upgrade the hardware of the body (Harisastri 2002):

As a result of the purificatory treatments followed by rejuvenation therapy done at the junctions of the seasons, the tissues become healthy, immunity and resistance are improved and the process of ageing is slowed down (Aṣṭāṅga Hṛdaya, Sūtra Sthāna, 7, 49 in Harisastri 2002).

Āyurveda points out that higher levels of health and well-being can be attained through such interventions. The role of the mind is cardinal in the process of successful ageing. One of the goals of Rasāyana is to keep one's mind supple and active in old age (Yadavji 1992):

The goal of Rasāyana or rejuvenation is not just to prolong life, but to also transform consciousness to a higher level of awareness (Ćaraka Saṃhitā, Cikitsā Sthāna, 1, 80 in Yadavji 1992)

Healthy ageing is an outcome of successful adaptation and evolution of the person as a whole. Emotional stability and cultivation of insight and awareness are as important as strengthening of tissues and immunity for healthy ageing. Āyurveda offers many interesting ideas, psychosomatic approaches and pharmacological interventions to facilitate successful ageing.

4.3 Physical and Mental Constitution

Āyurveda considers each individual to be unique, and consequently, a person-centred approach is advocated to not only curative medicine but also preventive and promotive interventions.

Variability between individuals stems from constitutional make-up. There are six types of constitutions in Āyurveda: (1) Racial Constitution, (2) Familial Constitution, (3) Geographical Constitution, (4) Temporal Constitution, (5) Age related Constitution and (6) Individual Specific Constitution (Ćaraka Saṃhitā, Indriya Sthāna, 1, 5 in Yadavji 1992). Certain characteristics of individuals may be specific to the race, family, geographical location, seasonal cycles and age. These are characteristics that are shared in common by the members of the group. Apart from that, there is the individual specific constitution which is of two types—the physical and the mental.

The physical constitution is subdivided into three broad categories which are further expanded to make seven phenotypes (Harisastri 2002). These seven types of physical constitution derive from the dominance of the three doṣas—*Vāta, Pitta, Kapha, Vātapitta, Vātakapha, Pittakapha*—and balance of all the three. The balanced constitution is the most healthy, and the dual combinations are the worst (Aṣṭāṅga Hṛdaya, Sūtra Sthāna, 1, 10 in Harisastri 2002).

Mental constitution is broadly of three types which when further subdivided makes at least sixteen categories (Yadavji 1992):

Mental constitution is broadly of three types - satva, rajas and tamas. … Out of these which can be subdivided into innumerable subtypes, there are 7 *satva* subtypes, 6 *rajas* subtypes and 3 *tamas* subtypes (Ćaraka Saṃhitā, Śārīra Sthāna, 4, 35–40 in Yadavji 1992)

The concept of the physical and mental constitution provides a framework to understand the variations between individuals. Though these categories help to generalise individual variations within limited classification, they actually serve as a flexible framework to pinpoint the peculiarities of an individual (see Chap. 9 for further details on this topic).

The *Ćaraka Saṃhitā* explicitly explains the interplay of physical and mental constitution in defining the health and well-being of an individual. The text clarifies that the three doṣas define the scope of health in the body while the three *guṇa* define the scope of well-being in the case of the mind (cited in Ćaraka Saṃhitā, Śārīra Sthāna, 4, 34 in Yadavji 1992).

The physical constitution is determined by the inherent balance of the three *doṣas*. While it is difficult to define and characterise the three *doṣas* within the scope of a short paper, it can be generally stated that the three *doṣas* actually represent the functional balance of the body. They are often erroneously translated as wind, bile and phlegm. They represent the totality of the anabolic and catabolic activities of the body (the concept of doṣas is deeply discussed also in Chaps. 3, 8, 9 and 10). Many attempts have been made to correlate these entities with functional expressions of the body. For example, *Vāta* is correlated with the nervous system, *Pitta* with the digestive and endocrine system and *Kapha* with immunity and the physical structures. In one sense, the *doṣas* represent the sum total of the exchange of matter and energy between the internal and external environment. *Vāta* represents the utilisation, *Pitta* the transformation and *Kapha* the preservation of energy. These processes generally tend to balance out each other. Depending on various factors including genetics and influences at the time of conception, the baseline gets fixed at different points in different individuals. As a result, there are individuals whose bodies tend to behave like energy conservers, others like energy transformers and still others like energy spenders. Thus, an individual with a *Kapha* constitution tends to preserve more energy than is spent. This trend has an impact on various physiological and psychological parameters and gives a calm, laid-back disposition to the individual who puts on weight and has a stable body. The *Vāta* constitution on the other hand tends to spend more energy than is conserved creating a psychological disposition characterised by thought diarrhoea, hyperactivity, anxiety and a physique that is poorly built and thin. The *Pitta* constitution tends to be transformative and hence has a creative mind and is very organised. At the physical level, they experience much heat and sweat in the body. The characteristics of different physical constitutions have been dealt elaborately in classical Ayurvedic texts. In recent times, attempts have been made to scientifically validate the Ayurvedic concept of *prakṛti* or physical constitution with encouraging results (Prasher et al. 2008; Bhushan et al. 2005; Patwardhan et al. 2006; Patwardhan and Bodeker 2008).

The combination of two and three doṣas creates additional personality types making seven broad categories in all. These combinations in different proportions create variations of personalities. The physical constitution cannot be changed, albeit it can be influenced by interventions at the time of conception (Yadavji 1992):

> The constitution formed at the time of conception becomes the basis for all the expressions of the individual. It is influenced by the sperm and ovum, the conditions in the uterus and

the diet and behaviour of the mother and the preponderance of the elements forming the fetus (Ćaraka Saṃhitā, Vimāna Sthāna, 4, 8–95 in Yadavji 1992)

Though it cannot be changed, physical constitution can be managed. The physical constitution sets the scope and limits for achieving higher levels of health. Assessment of the physical constitution is therefore the central component of personalised medicine in Āyurveda (Yadavji 1992; Harisastri 2002). In classical texts like *Ćaraka Saṃhitā* and *Aṣṭāṅga Hṛdaya*, constitution has been listed as one of the key factors to be checked to assess the disease and prescribe treatment. Physical constitution becomes therefore the reference point for working out a customised regimen for promotion and maintenance of health as well as for curative interventions.

The human personality is complex, and physical constitution cannot capture this complexity in totality. It is for this reason that Āyurveda discusses about racial constitution, familial constitution and so on and so forth. Two individuals with apparently similar physical constitution may have different expressions on account of racial and familial inheritance. The human being is multidimensional and so is the constitution. Apart from physical constitution, there is mental constitution that accounts for variability of one individual from another.

Mental constitution is broadly of three types depending on the nature of the mind to be aware, to be charged with emotion or just be ignorant. These three basic tendencies of the mind are known technically as *Satva, Rajas* and *Tamas*. They are known as *guṇa* or qualities, and these terms cannot be easily translated. We can only attempt to provide approximate definitions. *Satva* is a state of awareness of reality that brings calmness and quietude of the mind and an ability to respond to situations with composure. *Rajas*, on the other hand, is a very agitated state of the mind which distorts reality and leads the person to be overreactive to situations. *Tamas* is an indulgent and inert state of the mind characterised by lack of awareness leading to non-responsiveness to external situations. All the three are coexistent in everyone, and *Rajas* and *Tamas* within limits aid in expression of emotions and help in relaxation, withdrawal and rest.

The mind of different individuals can predominate in *Satva, Rajas* or *Tamas*, and thus, there are three broad mental types. However, there are many subtype variations within each category depending on the degree of dominance of the three *guṇa*. At least sixteen types of mental constitutions are described in the Ayurvedic texts (Yadavji 1992).

The complexity of the human personality stems from the dynamics or rather the interplay between the physical and mental constitution in the backdrop of the tendencies and traits inherited from one's race, family, place, time and age. The physical and mental constitution combines to create the unique individual. For example, a person who has a *Kapha* constitution physically can be *Sātvic* in mind whereas another person with the same physical constitution can be *Rajasic* in mind. An individual who has a *Rajasic* mental disposition and a *Pitta* constitution can be extremely explosive and violent, whereas one who has a *Sātvic* mental nature and a *Kapha* constitution can be extremely calm and peaceful.

A deep understanding of the complexity of human personality through the study of constitution enables the physician to understand the vulnerabilities and strengths of the individual from a medical point of view. The emotional tendencies, susceptibility to disease and ability to respond to stress and recover from illness are all anticipated with the help of analysis of the constitution of the individual.

According to Āyurveda, the body and mind make up a continuum, and so they influence each other profoundly. The relationship between the body and the mind is compared to that of ghee and an iron vessel. If ghee is poured into a hot iron vessel, then it becomes hot. Similarly, if hot ghee is poured into an iron vessel, the vessel also becomes hot. This is because the body and mind rest on an axis of continuity, and what happens in the body reflects on to the mind and vice versa (Cited in the commentary by Aruṇadatta on Aṣṭāṅga Hṛdaya, Sūtra Sthānaṃ, 1, 1 in Harisastri 2002).

For this reason, the *doṣas* which are seemingly physical constituents of the body are influenced and aggravated by psychological factors. For example, *Vāta* is associated with craving, depression and fear. *Pitta* is associated with anger and aggression (cited in Ćaraka Saṃhitā, Cikitsā Sthāna, 3, 115 in Yadavji 1992). On the other hand, Kapha is associated with calmness and joy (cited in Ćaraka Saṃhitā, Sūtra Sthāna 25, 40 in Yadavji 1992).

The physical constitution of an individual sets the limits, while the mind and the external environment sets the scope and potential for change and thereby enhancement of states of health. An individual with *Kapha* constitution cannot radically change his or her physical nature. But a *Kapha* type with *Tamasic* mind can transform into a *Rajasic* or *Satvic* type. So also with the other types of physical constitution. The chapter known as *Puruṣavicayaṃ Śārīraṃ* in *Ćaraka Saṃhitā* discusses about how the mind can be transformed into higher levels of consciousness with a predominance of *sattva* quality (Yadavji 1992):

> The cleansing of the mind is likened to the process of cleaning a dirty mirror. The satva quality of the mind can be enhanced by practice (Ćaraka Saṃhitā, Śārīra Sthāna 5, 13 in Yadavji 1992)

It is interesting to note that Āyurveda advises to allow the physiological urges of the body to express and not to interfere with them (Harisastri 2002). The physiological urges like flatus, faeces, urine, hunger, thirst and the like should not be provoked or suppressed. They should be allowed to express naturally. On the other hand, the emotional urges of the mind have to be checked (Harisastri 2002):

> One desirous of well being in this and other life must keep under control the emotional urges of greed, jealousy, aversion, competition and so on (Aṣṭāṅga Hṛdaya, Sūtra Sthāna 4, 24 in Harisastri 2002)

Emotional stability is itself synonymous with health. An emotionally stable person becomes very responsive and appropriate in actions, so much so that the physician par excellence is extolled as the one who eliminates the emotional instability of the mind (cited in Aṣṭāṅga Hṛdaya, Sūtra Sthāna 1, 1 in Harisastri 2002). In other words, it is by treating the mind of the person that wholeness is restored and established.

In a similar way, the environmental influences can be regulated to a great extent to optimise the expressions of the physical constitution. For instance, an individual of *Kapha* constitution can prevent imbalances by regulating exposure to environmental influences including food that can cause an imbalance of *Kapha*.

Āyurveda advises that a lifestyle should be adopted that is in tune with the peculiarities of the place as well as the season. Even the medicines used in treatment should be derived from the locality. It is a fundamental precept in Āyurveda that for the people living in a particular locality, the plants growing in that region are the most suited (Sharma 2012):

> The plants growing in the region where a person has been acclimatised is best suited for that individual (Aṣṭāṅga Saṃgraha, Sūtra Sthāna 23, 95 in Sharma 2012)

The interplay of the body and the mind is the basis for health as well as disease. In that sense, the Ayurvedic approach to management of health is psychosomatic in its outlook. Āyurveda distinguishes between the mind and the body, which are both considered as material and different from the self. The mind is subtle, and the body is gross. In spite of the differences, the body and mind are continuous and flow into each other. They cannot function without influencing one another or rather they cannot function in isolation. The harmony between body and mind is the foundation for good health, and body-mind conflicts are in the background of majority of diseases. Understanding physical and mental constitution provides a framework to understand the interactions of body and mind in each individual and to work out a strategy to establish harmony. To put it in one phrase, the Ayurvedic approach to good health is to 'manage the body and to transform the mind'. There is a limit to changing the nature of the body once constitution is formed at the time of conception. One has to learn to manage the body by adopting appropriate lifestyle modifications. On the other hand, there is greater scope for influencing and transforming mental states, and with training, it is possible to attain emotional stability and mental well-being that can enable the individual to cope with physical and environmental limitations in the most effective manner.

4.4 The Person-Centred Approach to Health Care

Āyurveda offers an approach to health care that aims to achieve longevity and healthy ageing. The constitution of the individual sets non-negotiable limits to enhance health, and therefore a great deal of effort has been focused on prenatal and postnatal interventions to develop a healthy constitution. Living to a ripe old age in the pink of health is an outcome of a life that is established in a healthy lifestyle. Health is a dynamic process that adapts to external circumstances and evolves to higher levels of expression. The physical and mental constitution of the individual sets the scope for each individual to discover the roadmap to attain the highest peak of health that can be attained given the limitations of the constitution and the environment in which the person is embedded.

4.5 Conclusion

Āyurveda is the knowledge of life and much more than a medical system. Its primary focus is on longevity and healthy ageing. Curing diseases is only one of the means to work towards the target of higher levels of health. Health is visualised as a dynamic, adaptive and evolutionary process that has to be facilitated through interventions derived from a proper understanding of the constitution of the individual and the environmental matrix. To sum up, the approach of Āyurveda is echoed in the words of Osler: 'The good physician treats the disease, the great physician treats the person with the disease'. Āyurveda is concerned with the well-being of the person, known as *Karma Puruṣa*, and the knowledge of Āyurveda has been revealed for the sake of this person struggling to find his way up the ladder of healthy existence.

References

Bhushan, P., Kalpana, J., & Arvind, C. (2005). Classification of human population based on HLA gene polymorphism and the concept of Prakriti in Āyurveda. *Journal of Alternative and Complementary Medicine, 11*, 349–353.

Harisastri, P. V. (Ed.). (2002). *Ashtanga Hridayam*. Varanasi: Chaukhambha Orientalia.

Patwardhan, B., & Bodeker, G. (2008). Ayurvedic genomics: Establishing a genetic basis for mindbody typologies. *Journal of Alternative and Complementary Medicine, 214*, 571–576.

Patwardhan, B., Joshi, K., & Ghodke, Y. (2006). Genetic basis to concept of Prakriti. *Current Science, 90*, 896.

Prasher, B., Negi, S., Aggarwal, S., Mandal, A. K., Sethi, T. P., Deshmukh, S. R., et al. (2008). Whole genome expression and biochemical correlates of extreme constitutional types defined in Āyurveda. *Journal of Translational Medicine, 6*, 48.

Sahebrao, G. N. (2009). *Vedic philosophy of values*. New Delhi: Northern Book Centre.

Sharma, S. (Ed.). (2012). *Ashtanga Sangraha*. Varanasi: Chaukhambha Sanskrit Series Office.

Yadavji, T. A. (Ed.). (1980). *Suśruta Samhita*. Varanasi: Chaukhambha Orientalia.

Yadavji, T. A. (Ed.). (1992). *Ćaraka Samhita*. New Delhi: Munshilal Manoharlal Publishers Pvt. Ltd.

Chapter 5
Determinants of Health and Well-Being in Āyurveda

A.N. Narayanan Nambi

5.1 Introduction

Eastern traditional medicine is one of the most sophisticated indigenous systems. It holds an unbroken tradition spanning more than five millennia. Though this medical heritage is many centuries old, even today millions of people in villages, towns, and cities across eastern countries depend upon it for their daily healthcare needs. All these indigenous systems hold two kinds of tradition: folk and structured. Folk tradition encompasses diverse practices, in which modifications were introduced from time to time according to the changing needs of the society. The structured systems of knowledge, like Āyurveda and Siddha, try instead to find the rationality of each practice and record it in encrypted form, totally differing in this respect from the folk tradition. While the former focuses on the nature-man relationship, the latter focuses on the man-self relationship. Both systems survived over millennia, assimilated all the possible variations of human nature, and projected possibilities for better survival and balance.

It is impossible to understand any system without the knowledge of its origin. In biological systems, there is a deep unity between origin, structure, and function. As aptly stated by the biologist Theodosius Dobzhansky (quoted in Ramachandran 2010, p. 14):

> Nothing in biology makes sense except in the light of evolution.

As there is a close link between origin, structure, and functions in all biological systems, there is an inseparable link between health and healing. From this

A.N. Narayanan Nambi (✉)
SNA Oushadhasala Pvt. Ltd, Thrissur, Kerala, India
e-mail: drnambi@hotmail.com

A. Morandi and A.N. Narayanan Nambi (eds.), *An Integrated View of Health and Well-being*, Cross-Cultural Advancements in Positive Psychology 5, DOI 10.1007/978-94-007-6689-1_5,

perspective, as Gerald Larson suggested, South Asian medical theory and practice can offer new and useful insights:

> What is of importance in traditional medicine....is a way of valuing and a way of conceptualizing "disease" and "illness" that is interestingly different from our own and that is not at all incompatible with the rigorous precision of modern scientific methodology. (Larson 1993, p. 104)

5.2 The Pursuit for Health

"Health" not only refers to a biological condition (Halfbass 1991). It rather reflects a broader frame which includes aspects such as freedom from incapacitation, vitality for successful action, and feeling of well-being. Health care should be related to such a broader framework, encompassing traditional and contemporary systems of medicine, preventive routines and treatment methods, and social issues such as the economics of health insurance (as highlighted in Chap. 3 of this volume). Unfortunately, the term health care has been very much reduced to just illness care by contemporary biomedicine, where the medical intervention is undertaken after the development of illness, neglecting the person's inherent vitality and immunity as well as the possibility to diagnose or prevent potential problems (Chap. 3 of this volume provides a detailed description of this current trend). Āyurveda instead emphasizes the importance of preventive methods and fosters health as a positive state, providing a complementary view to the more crisis-oriented self-managing model. While the biomedical model gives most of its attention to the theory and treatment of disease, Āyurveda shows more concern for the active development of health (see Chap. 10 for further discussion of this topic).

In the preamble to the Constitution of the World Health Organization, health is defined as:

> ...a state of complete physical, mental, and social well-being and not merely the absence of disease or infirmity (quoted in Caplan et al. 1981)

This definition recognizes the multiple domains of human life in which health is important and regards health as a positive state, not merely as a concept whose meaning is established in relation to illness, disability, or sickness. Total well-being or perfect health is generally thought to be a utopian concept. Though we think of health in various dimensions, medical science mostly limits it to the physical and mental aspects, often neglecting the complex web of relationship existing among all living systems. In fact, individuals are offered a wide range of possibilities to maintain perfect health and functioning, thanks to their ceaseless interaction with the environment and their responses to the various sociocultural demands.

5.3 The Conceptual Core of Āyurveda

It has been correctly told that Āyurveda is the knowledge (*veda*) of life (*āyu*), but the literal meaning of the word *āyu* implies something that is getting naturally and progressively diminished. As a living being is constituted not merely by body but also by senses (*indriyas*), mind (*manas*), and Self or Consciousness (*ātma*), this conceptualization of *āyu* encompasses all these components. Since birth, all these components undergo modifications and reformations, except *ātma*, the unchanging and eternal consciousness principle that is hosted in individuals throughout their life. Hence, *āyu* is also named as *dhāri* that literally stems from the word *dhāraṇa* (to hold the *ātman*). The period of *ātma's* sojourn in the body is defined as *jīvita* or lifespan. Since *ātman* is imperishable, it is also called *nityaga*, and since it endures, it is also named *anubandha* (Ćaraka Saṃhitā, Suthrasthana 1, 42 in Brahmanad Tripathi 1997).

Since *āyu* is progressive and deteriorative by nature, the only way to enjoy life at its maximum is through maintaining an adequate balance in the complexity of the system. Āyurveda provides a description of the interaction between the *pro-āyu* (*āyushaṣya*) and *against-āyu* (*anāyuṣhya*), assuming that when such knowledge gets translated into action, it can be fruitfully used in health-related practices. To this purpose Āyurveda proposes specific *śasana* or canons of right and wrong action and thought. Only the repeated practice of correct behaviors and activities can bring benefits to a person as individual or to the society at large. However, behaviors and activities are outcomes of the mind work, which allows for correct understanding of the situation, also based on associations with previous experience – *anumāna* or inference. This allows the formation of a web of cause/effect relationships between the individual and the environment. Knowledge is meaningless without the basic understanding of this relationship network, acquired with the help of *anumāna* (inference) of the cycle of cause and effect.

The ultimate aim of Āyurveda as *śāstra* (science) is to know all possible causes and effects that come into play in both the conditions of wellness and illness. Only by understanding its causes, a disease can be controlled; similarly, only by knowing the causes of health, it may be maintained and pursued. A large amount of information concerning these processes was collected by the ancient scholars on the basis of direct perception (*Pratyakṣa*) as well as inferences, tested by time and named as *aptopadeśa* or *āgama*. These terms refer to peculiar psychological features: though everyone can exert direct perception and perform inference, the effectiveness of this process depends on the refinement of sense organs and on the stability of mind. People characterized by a condition of optimal functioning and balance are called as *āpta*, and their knowledge is named as *āpta upadeśa*, meaning that it can transcend time and space in its applications.

5.4 Theories of Existence of Life

With the help of the three knowledge forms (*Pramāna*), namely, *Pratyakṣa*, *Anumāna*, and *Āptopadeśa*, the existence of life is explained by Ācharya Suśruta through the acknowledgement of six possible existences of life:

Swabhāvam éswaram kālam yadruccham niyatim thadha.
Pariṇāmam ca manyanthe prakṛutim pradhu darśinah (Suśruta Saṃhitā, Sūtra Sthāna 1, 11 in Laxmidhar Dwivedi 1998)

1. *Swabhāva* – by its nature
2. *Ēśwara* – by divine support
3. *Kāla* – by time
4. *Yadrucchā* – by uncertainty
5. *Niyati* – by law
6. *Pariṇāma* – by evolution

The scholars of Āyurveda commonly accepted *swabhāva* as the main cause of existence, though they did not negate the others. This primacy of nature makes the definition of life universally valid in its outlook, as per Acharya Ćaraka:

So ayamāyurvedah śāśwato nirdiśyate anāditwat, swabhāva samsiddha lakshaṇatwat, bhāva swabhāva nityatwat ca. (Ćaraka Saṃhitā, Sūtra Sthāna 30, 27 in Brahmanad Tripathi 1997)

(Ayurveda is said to be eternally continuous because of its beginningless-ness, the characters of entities having been determined by universal nature and the characters of substances being eternal).

Within the perspective of Āyurveda, the following sections will illustrate the various realms of the body in all possible levels and how they are connected in an integrated and interrelated system.

5.5 Understanding the Body

In Indian philosophy each body is not singular; rather, it is a combination of three bodies: the *gross body* (*Sthūla śarīra*), the one that is perceived by our senses, nourished by food; the *subtle body* (*Sūkṣma śarīra)*, the one that cannot be perceived by the senses but it is known to each one of us, for example, I know whether I am hungry or angry but others may not know it till I express it through my gross body; and the *causal body* (*Kāraṇa śarīra*), which is the seat of all our inherent tendencies (*vāsanas*) and the cause for the other bodies.

5.5.1 *The Three Bodies and Their Relationship*

Gross body is made up of five fundamental elements: space, air, fire, water, and earth, as the outcome of the progressive grossification (*Panjīkaraṇa*) of reality (see Chaps. 3 and 10 for an overview of the conceptualization of reality and its evolution in Indian tradition). This evolved body will dissolve back at the time of death and will disintegrate into fundamental elements. Through this body, we experience joy and sorrow. It temporarily ceases its functioning during sleep and permanently at the time of death.

Subtle body, which pervades the gross body, is made up of a nascent form of fundamental elements (*tanmātra*) that cannot be perceived by senses. We cannot see other's mind neither our own, yet we are aware of the thoughts occurring in our mind. This subtle body consists of 17 components: five sensory organs of perception (sound, touch, vision, taste, smell), five organs of action (speech, hands, legs, excretory, and reproductive organs), five vital principles or *prāṇas* (*Samāna, Vyāna, Udāna, Prāṇa, Apāna*), the mind (*Manas*), and the intellect (*Buddhi*).

Causal body is the subtlest of three bodies. It pervades the other two and it is the repository for all our inherent tendencies and lack of knowledge. It cannot be explained and experienced, and it is carried from birth to birth (Tejomayananda 2000).

When the consciousness identifies itself with the gross body, it manifests as the awakener that enjoys a wakened world and its myriad experiences. The same when withdrawing from the gross body, it identifies with the subtle body. In this condition, it manifests itself as the dreamer experiencing the dream world. Similarly, withdrawing from the gross and subtle bodies and identifying with the causal body, it functions as a deep-sleeper who undergoes a homogeneous experience of void. In addition to the three stages mentioned above, there is another stage which is termed as "death" – a state of absolute cessation of all experiences. Hence, its antonym (of death), the "*life*" is a stream of experiences, each of them becoming "unit of life" just as a single brick in a wall. Just as the strength and the weakness of the wall depends upon the quality and the texture of the bricks constituting it, the type of experiences that individuals undergo shall determine the character and temperament of their life. If their experiences are happy, their life is happy, and if they are miserable, their life is also miserable.

5.6 Experience and Life

An individual derives his experience from receiving and responding to various stimuli from the external world. An experience therefore is constituted by the following three entities:

The experiencer (who is experiencing) – the subject
The experienced (i.e., the outcome of experience) – the object
The experiencing – the relationship between the subject and the object

The primary field of enquiry among the eastern sages was the "experiencer," whereas that of western scientists is the "experienced." The aim of the eastern sages was to show the possibility to optimally develop the inner personality, in order to develop independence from the changing environment and occurrences of the

Disposition	Attributes	Outcome
Brahmaṇa (Spiritual)	*Ātma* (Consciousness)	*Mokṣha* (Salvation)
Kṣhatriya (Intellectual)	*Buddhi* (Intelligence)	*Dharma* (Righteousness)
Vaiśya (Psychological)	*Manas* (Mind)	*Kāma* (Desire)
Sūdra (Physical)	*Śarira* (Body)	*Artha* (Resources)

Fig. 5.1 The four-level categorization of personal dimensions and related outcomes

world. The result of this process is the elevation of the *standard of life*. On the other hand, western scientists try to make the world a better place to living, in an attempt to raise the *standard of living*.

5.6.1 Realms of Experience

The analysis of the experience led the Indian scholars to conclude that it emanates from different levels within the person, all of them unique in themselves. It was also acknowledged that the four different dimensions or dispositions – physical, psychological, intellectual, and spiritual – work together in a human being even though he himself may not able to comprehend it (Fig. 5.1). When a subject comes in contact with an object, it does so, not as an integrated whole but with four distinct personalities as it were from four layers of the person. Four differently constituted entities, each having its own demands and values, awake at the challenge of every situation created by an object or being, or thrust upon to experience it.

Thus every moment, in each of our experiences, four different constituents are at work within us, in order to comprehend the situation and earn the treasure of the experience. When these four different powers – behaving as dichotomous strangers from different realms, each characterized by different values and demands – come together to enjoy any given object or situation, this event will invariably bring satisfaction to one at varying degrees and dissatisfaction to the other three. This confusion of personalities within ourselves creates a tragic chaotic condition which disturbs peace and tranquility; the eternal human search for joy and happiness, thrust for perfection, and sound health get blasted and push individuals to the edge of restlessness, desperation, and subsequently ill-health. In his eternal search for happiness, tranquility, and peace, individuals pursue new occasions to experience a more perfect and complete well-being by changing the arrangement of things and circumstances, in the ultimate hope that they may get eternal peace and happiness to the fullest and deepest extent.

The ancient sages of health-care systems knew very well these desperate conditions, into which humans are helplessly pushed by the circumstances, and they preached solutions by which individuals could efficiently and fruitfully integrate all the distinct four personalities within themselves and find a condition conducive to happiness with lesser efforts (Chinmayananda 2002).

5.6.2 Dispositions, Attributes, and Outcomes

According to Indian system of knowledge, it is possible to distinguish between four basic personalities, which are manifestations based on the qualities and actions they perform, as summarized in Fig. 5.1. This is portrayed in detail in Bhagavad Gita:

> *Chāturvarṇyam mayā sṛuṣtam guṇakarmavibhāgaśah* (Bhāgavad Gita, IV/13 in Swami Rama 1998)
> (I have created the four fold classification on the basis of their qualities and actions)

Unfortunately these grouping are well-known to western readers as the caste system that characterized Indian society, but they were originally meant to explain the various kinds of individuals according to their nature in qualities and actions. Here, we consider these four groups as useful concepts to explain the nature of humans and their opportunity to grow further or to move forward (from *Rajasic* or *Tamasic* towards absolute *Satwa* – see Chap. 4 for a detailed analysis of these concepts).

The physical entity of a living being may be termed as *Śūdra* (literally a lower class in the cast system, devoted to manual jobs), and it refers to the primitive disposition. The *Śūdra* derives the resources for his survival from the other three groups. His values are essentially mundane in character.

The psychological entity, which is in an elevated status compared with *Śūdra*, enjoys the desires and aesthetics in nature and may be termed as the *Vaiśya* (which literally means the business community). It holds its own values and virtues to be adhered to in life.

Further, the intellectual disposition can be designated as a still higher class, the *Kṣatriya* (literally the class of community of rulers), whose values are broader in vision and are based on *dharma*.

Lastly, we reach the supreme personality of the *Brahmaṇa* (which literally means the community of priests, whose ultimate aim in life is the attainment of *mokṣa* or salvation or eternal bliss). *Brahmaṇa* means who knows *Brahma* – the ultimate truth. In its search for the ultimate truth, this disposition becomes identified with the infinite, whose boundaries are nowhere and whose center is everywhere.

5.7 The Health Status

In the light of the above discussed concepts, the ancient Āyurvedic scholars – especially Ćaraka – propagated that the pathological disturbance of the fundamental principles (*doṣa*) creates morbidity, whereas the balancing of the same to normalcy creates health:

> *Vikāro dhātu vaiṣamyam Sāmyam prakṛutiruchate* (Ćaraka Saṃhitā, Sūtra Sthāna 9, 4 in Brahmanad Tripathi 1997)

A similarly normative doctrine is exemplified by Georg Canguilhem (1989), who uses the terms "health" and "disease" as normative terms. Health means that a person functions well and disease makes him/her function badly:

> Man feels in good health - what is health itself - only when he feels more than normal - that is, adapted to the environment and its demands. - but normative, capable of following new norms of life....for man health is a feeling of assurance in life to which no limit is fixed. *Valere*, from which value derives, means to be in good health in Latin. Health is a way of tackling existence as one feels that one is not only possessor or bearer but also, if necessary, creator of value, and establisher of vital norms (Canguilhem 1989, p. 200)

In an elaborative sense, a healthy individual is defined in Āyurveda as the *swastha* expected to have balance in humors (*doṣa*), structural tissues (*dhātu*), excretory functions (*mala*), and digestive capacity and the tranquility of consciousness (*Ātman*), mind (*Manas*), and senses (*Indriya*).

> *Sama doṣa samāgnisca samadhātu malakriyah*
> *Prasannātmendriya manah swastha etyabhidīyate...*
> (Suśruta Saṃhitā, Sūtra Sthāna 15, 41 in Laxmidhar Dwivedi 1998)

A biological perspective professed by Christopher Boorse (1977) also expressed the same concept, defining health as "functional normality." This perspective uses the terms "health" and "disease" as descriptive, neutral-value terms. To say that a person or an organ or system is healthy means that its functions are normal; to say it is diseased means that its functions are abnormal, with biostatistical data providing the criteria of normality:

> ... diseases are internal states that depress a functional ability below species-typical levels. Health as freedom from disease is then statistical normality of function, i.e., the ability to perform all typical physiological functions with at least typical efficiency (Christopher Boorse 1977, p. 542)

Hence, the doyens in Āyurveda emphasize a much wider framework within which to analyze the whole process which is said to be the primordial cause of all disease.

5.8 A Framework to Understand Health and Its Alterations

Figure 5.2 illustrates a model of health that encompasses not merely the body but the person's multiple attributes, including responses towards external environment. It deals with the complete pattern of interactions within the individual and towards the external environments as well as its ultimate balance. While the "balance" is only one, "imbalances" are innumerable, and they comprise all possible deviations from balance and their probable outcomes. In particular, at the level of actions, imbalances can be due to an excess, an insufficiency, or an improper performance of action.

The advantage of this framework is that it can transcend all geographical, cultural, religious, and racial discriminations and can represent human entity as a

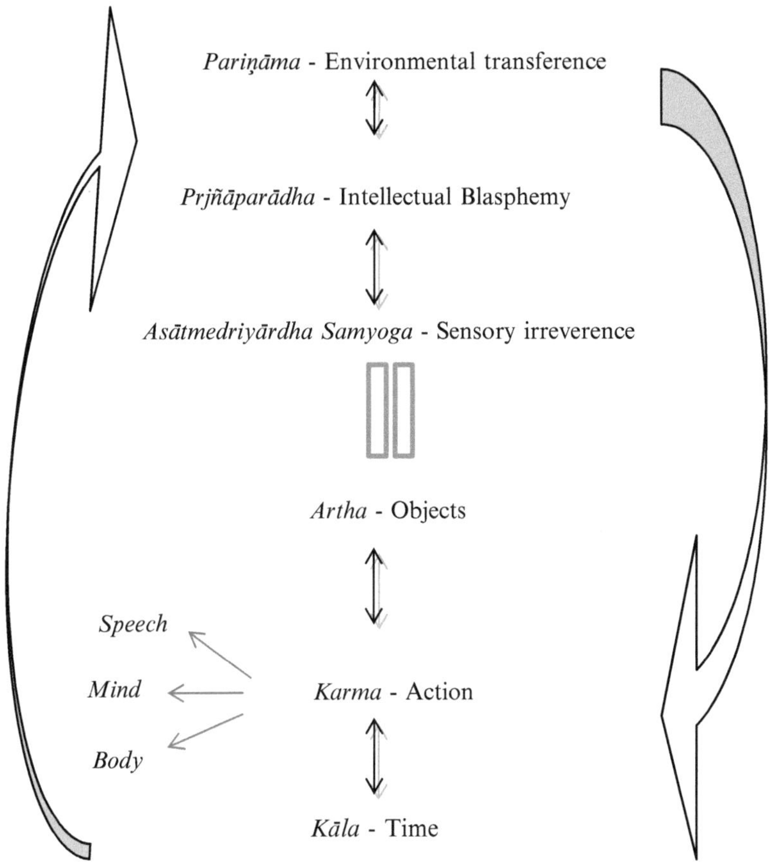

Fig. 5.2 Factors contributing to the alterations of health and well-being

whole, observing its inherent universal tendencies. Moreover, any philosophical system can find place within it. This idea is universal in it its outlook and it is suggestive of a new vision of health.

5.8.1 Theory of Inherent Tendencies (Asātmedriyārtha Samyoga)

According to Āyurveda, similarity increases similarity. Thus desires, habits, and actions have the potential to shape the character of an individual. We ultimately become what we desire, think, eat, and do. The activities we perform towards outside are sensorial, and they can be of two types: perceptive and reactive. Perceptive activities are based on the perceptive senses – eyes, ears, nose, tongue, and skin – which

Fig. 5.3 Sense organs and their objects

Sense Organs	Objects
Eyes	*Rūpa* (Sight)
Nose	*Gandha* (Smell)
Tongue	*Rasa* (Taste)
Skin	*Sparśa* (Touch)
Ears	*Śabda* (Sound)

make contact with the external environment and collect the information from the objects. The actions of the senses are limited in terms of site, range, as well as performance, and they are controlled and regulated by *Manas* (mind) and *Buddhi* (intellect). Reactive activities are based on the reactive senses that actively express themselves through specific organs: tongue (by the act of speech), hands, legs, and excretory and reproductive organs. Again, these are structurally bounded and controlled by mind and intellect. Excessive, decreased, or abnormal use of them will disturb the balance, resulting in ill-health. For example, eyes are the sense to see and they collect vision related information. But if we over exert them, for example, sitting in front of computers for long hours without break, it will result in eye dryness, an alteration in their physiology. Since senses are limited in site, range, and performance within an organ of perception, the violation of these limits leads to the development of a diseased condition or at least to a deviation from the state of wellbeing. If the individual is able to follow his own internal resonance defined by multiple determinants, he will get balanced.

In sensory perception, the action takes place when the stimuli received from outside under the limited domain of sense organs reach the mind. Hence, it is important to define the determinants involved in this process: object of sense, organ of sense, presence of mind, and sensory intelligence.

Sense Objects: All the senses are bound to their own objects, and they are exclusive in nature. One sense cannot accept the object specific of another sense, and each one has an optimal range of perception which depends on the organ of sense and its constitution. Beyond that range, it cannot perceive. For example, a continuous highly illuminated light will hamper the vision.

Sense Organs: These are the structural entities of the body that participate in the act of perception. However, the whole act of comprehending the perception is not limited to a single organ, rather involving a chain of structures which collectively carry out the process. If during the continuous flow of perception, any of the constituents become damaged or unable to perform correctly, it becomes a determinant of alteration of health (Fig. 5.3).

Mind: Mind (*Manas*) is the most crucial component in the whole activity of perception, and its lack of participation creates absence of information. Hence again, the status of mind at its purest form will bring the best out of the perception process. Āyurveda recommends purity of mind in the sense that it has not to be clouded with emotions, such as anger, grief, or anger.

Sensory Intelligence: The intelligence represents the inherent ergonomic system which regulates the sense organs. It is also a crucial element, and any damage to it causes a variety of health problems.

5.8.2 Theory of Sin Against Wisdom (Prjñāparādha)

Asian philosophies believe that living beings have the inner capacity to follow the suggestions and messages arising from their innermost core, in order to be guided in achieving life's goals. This capacity may be shadowed by individual tendencies and inclinations, resulting in mistakes in life which are one of the root causes for human miseries. This process is called *Prjñāparādha*; here the word "*Prjñā*" refers to the inner source from where the messages originate, while *aparādha* refers to negligence or infringement.

The mind always develops thoughts and desires which in turn create illusions of separation. For example, the Indian philosophical system believes that death is only a transient change of shelter for the imperishable *Ātman*. However, mind is always ignorant of this true identity and, due to its attachment to the current life that it considers as unique, it develops the fear of death. So mind acts through its desire. It will grasp and get attached to pleasant experiences as a way to avoid changes that are seen as a manifestation of separation, of death. Analogously, through unhealthy aversions from negative experiences, the mind pushes away those experiences in order to escape the associated changes. In this way desire and aversion become the root cause for many diseases, if acted out without taking due consideration of *buddhi*, also named as *Prjñā* in Āyurvedic literature. But if guided by inner wisdom, the fruit of action will be true and genuine. The proximity with inner or external events, phenomena, or entities – be it a pathogen or an emotion or a thought form – allows for potentially fruitful exchanges, which are very vital for an organism as an open system. This fosters a bio-moral-environmental transaction, based on the interrelationship of all things and all possible interactions at every level. Any deviation from this will obstruct the interrelationship, which in turn can generate an imbalance in the system either sooner or later.

Prjñāparāda is thus a form of intransigence or inability, or desire for a difference or separateness as microcosm, with the illusory aim to remain in the state of harmony.

Āyurveda, in order to avoid such situations, focuses on daily regimen as a means of balancing the mind and focusing desire through continuous repetitive behaviors known as rituals. Daily regimen prescribes behaviors beyond desire or aversion in terms of diet, exercise, routine prayers, and restrictions in life-style activities, including sexual life. These practices facilitate the natural distancing from unhealthy desires and aversions, and their consequences, bringing the individual microcosm back into its inner balance or harmony. Daily, seasonal, or social regimens are designed to ensure optimization in the bio-moral-environmental transactions, no matter whether body or mind may like or dislike the whole act.

5.8.3 Theory of Environmental Transference (Pariṇāma)

As life originates and develops, it acts as an open system not separated from the environment, being connected with it by the influx and efflux of nutritional materials and waste products. This open system maintains a steady concentration of its constituents, given their constant formation as well as the continuous exchange and interplay of molecules and chemical groupings in virtually all body tissues and fluids. The apparent stability and permanency of the living organism is the result of a careful balancing between building up and breaking down processes in a steady state, even though material is constantly passing into and out of the system. The steady state is stable thanks to a long sequence of reactions, like what happens in the metabolic processes of the living cell. Slight modifications in the reservoirs, in the reaction rates, or at the beginning or end of the reaction chain have little disturbing effect on the concentration of substances in the reaction chain.

As nature changes in time, human body also expresses its changes as an open system. Body exhibits willingness to rearrange through alterations in the qualities of principles (*doṣa*) manifesting a subclinical morbidity. Under customary circumstances, this alteration is balanced by various feedback mechanisms and is never been noticed. Balance is achieved through two factors: (a) reduction of the contrast between etiological factors and individual status (*doṣa*) and (b) coherence between physiological principles (*doṣa*) and structural components (*dhātu*) (Ćaraka Saṃhitā, Nidanasthana, 4, 4 in Brahmanad Tripathi 1997).

Changes in seasons and their influences on body systems may be taken as an example. In normalcy, human body is exposed to the nature's changes since birth, and it will adapt to them in time. But if alterations take place in the natural pattern of environmental changes, the body will need substantial efforts to understand them and to adjust to the anomalous situation. Three varieties of change may occur: hyper-expression of nature (e.g., flood instead of rain), hypo-expression of nature (e.g., drought instead of rain), or improper expression of nature (e.g., untimely seasons).

From this perspective, all expressions of nature can be transposed in terms of unexpected experiences in day-to-day life at the level of the social and cultural contexts. Whatever may be the external factors or systems that get altered, Āyurveda recommends to check the balance of principles (*doṣa*), structural tissues (*dhātu*), and waste products (*mala*) at the individual level, which define vital harmony and well-being.

In line with these concepts, Claude Bernard, working in the nineteenth-century climate of Lamarck's and Darwin's evolutionary theories, regarded disease as a result of an organism's failure to adapt to environmental insults (Dubos 1979).

Similarly, Brody and Sobel's systems theory of health endorses Dubos' position according to which

> states of health or disease are the expression of the success or failure experienced by an organism in its effort to respond adaptively to environmental challenges. (Brody and Sobel 1979, p. 93).

The systems theory view of health incorporates various levels or domains, through which information flows in a pattern of feedback loops. Brody and Sobel summarize the concept of health as

> the ability of a system (i.e., cell, organism, family, society) to respond adaptively to a wide variety of environmental challenges (i.e. physical, chemical, infectious, psychological, social). (Brody and Sobel 1979, p. 91)

5.9 Conclusion

The ancient wisdom of Āyurveda through its intricate analysis of *Sthūla śarīra*, *Sūkṣma śarīra*, and *Kāraṇa śarīra* highlighted the subtle relationship among all the possible levels of human being, understood the possibilities of human being's multiplicity of experiences, and forecasted their possible outcomes as health and miseries. By formalizing the theory of inherent tendencies, of sin against wisdom, and of environmental transference, it vividly elucidates the existence of human beings both in the individual and in the collective dimension. In particular, the theory of inherent tendencies provides a core description of human existence and behavior, whose validity can be ascertained across time and cultures. Moreover, Āyurveda emphasizes the importance of rituals not merely as a religious doctrine or dogma but as a tool or vehicle to connect microcosm to macrocosm rather naturally than mechanically. These areas surely require further study and research, since their potential for application – largely proved by the uninterrupted and effective use of Āyurveda across millennia in the Indian subcontinent – can provide new insights for the development of a more integrated view of health that can overcome cultural boundaries.

References

Boorse, C. (1977). Health as a theoretical concept. *Philosophy of Science, 44*, 542.

Brahmanad Tripathi. (1997). *Ćaraka Samhitha Suthrasthana Ch.1/42*. Varanasi: Chowkhambha Sanskrit Pratisthan.

Brody, H., & Sobel, D. S. (1979). A systems view of health and disease. In D. S. Sobel (Ed.), *Ways of health: Holistic approaches to ancient and contemporary medicine*. New York/London: Harcourt Brace Jovanovich.

Canguilhem, G. (1989). *On the normal and the pathological* (C. R. Fawcett, English Trans.). New York: Zone Books.

Caplan, A. L., et al. (1981). Constitution of the World Health Organization. In A. L. Caplan, H. T. Engelhardt Jr., & J. J. McCartney (Eds.), *Concepts of health and disease, interdisciplinary perspectives* (p. 83). Reading: Addison-Wesley.

Dubos, R. (1979). Hippocrates in modern dress. In D. S. Sobel (Ed.), *Ways of health: Holistic approaches to ancient and contemporary medicine*. New York/London: Harcourt Brace Jovanovich.

Halfbass, W. (1991). *Tradition and reflection: Explorations in Indian thought*. Albany: State University of New York Press.

Larson, G. J. (1993). Āyurveda and the Hindu philosophical systems. In T. P. Kasulis, R. T. Ames, & W. Dissanayake W (Eds.), *Self as body in Asian theory and practice*. Albany: State University of New York Press. (Originally published in Philosophy East and West. 37, July 1987)

Laxmidhar Dwivedi. (Ed.). (1998). *Sushrutha Samhitha*. Varanasi: Chowkhamba Sanskrit Series Office.

Ramachandran, V. S. (2010). *Overview. The tell-tale brain, unlocking the mystery of human nature*. Delhi: Random House India.

Swami Chinmayananda. (2002). *Kindle life*. Mumbai: Chinmaya Mission Trust.

Swami Rama. (1998). *Perennial psychology of the Bhagavat Gita*. Honesdale, Pennsylvania, USA: The Himalayan International Institute.

Tejomayananda. (2000). *Commentary on Tatwa bodhah of Sri Adi Sankaracharya*. Mumbai: Chinmaya Mission Trust.

Chapter 6
The Role of Social Rituals in Well-Being

P.R. Krishna Kumar

6.1 Introduction

Rituals are part and parcel of the daily life of people in the cultural traditions of India. So much so that even routine activities have been ritualized. From simple acts like salutation, eating, and bathing to complex temple ceremonies, rituals permeate almost all aspects of the life of the people of India. Ritualization represents an attempt to structure and regulate behavior, so that an environment and atmosphere conducive to well-being is maintained in the inner life of the individual and the outer life of society at large. The dictum "social order has its roots in rituals" seems to be the underlying principle behind the ritualization of human behavior (cited in Vishnusahasranama 2010). Regulated and ritualized behavior is considered to be the source of law and order, or rather harmony in the inner and outer life of human beings.

6.2 Defining Rituals

A fundamental principle that characterizes the Indian approach to life is that happiness or well-being is an outcome of a righteous life, a life that is grounded in *dharma*.

Dharma is a difficult word to translate, and literally it means any action that leads to long-term stability and sustainability of any undertaking in the world. In a restricted sense, dharma can be equated to law and order, morality, and ethics. The classical texts of Āyurveda proclaim that happiness or well-being cannot be obtained without adherence to *dharma* (Harisastri 2002):

> The actions of all beings are aimed to achieve happiness. Happiness cannot be obtained without dharma and hence one should adhere to dharma (Aṣṭāṅga Hṛdaya, Sūtra Sthāna, II, 20 in Harisastri 2002)

P.R.K. Kumar (✉)
Arya Vaidya Pharmacy, Coimbatore, Tamil Nadu, India
e-mail: aniyancbe@yahoo.com

A. Morandi and A.N. Narayanan Nambi (eds.), *An Integrated View of Health and Well-being*, Cross-Cultural Advancements in Positive Psychology 5, DOI 10.1007/978-94-007-6689-1_6,

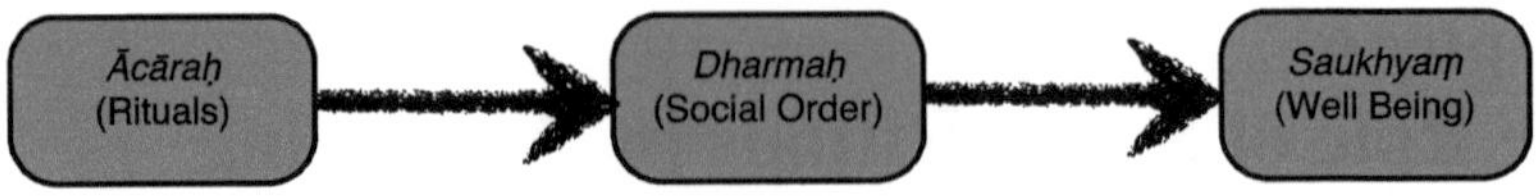

Fig. 6.1 Rituals and well-being. This diagram shows the relationship between rituals (ācāra) and well-being (saukhya). It illustrates the point that rituals help in achieving well-being through the agency of dharma or social order

(See Fig. 6.1) Hence, a blessed life has three dimensions: life, health, and well-being; āyurārogyasaukhyaṃ is a three-word summary indicating quality of life embracing life span, health, and well-being, made popular through a verse in the devotional poem *Nārāyaṇīyaṃ* composed in praise of Lord *Viṣhṇu.*

The purpose of rituals therefore is to establish dharma or harmony in human society, which in turn leads to well-being and happiness. *Vāgbhaṭa* in his *Aṣṭāṅga Hṛdaya Saṃhitā* makes this connection explicitly when he says:

> This is the proper conduct in a nut shell and compliance with these guidelines helps one to attain life, health, prosperity, fame and eternal realms of experience (Aṣṭāṅga Hṛdaya Saṃhitā, Sutra Sthana, 2, 48 in Harisastri 2002)

In other words, *ācāra* impacts different dimensions of well-being: security of life, security of health, standards of living, social recognition, and secure future.

The word *ācāra* cannot be exactly translated as ritual. It means good conduct and behavior or rather formal behavior. Rituals and ritualized behavior come within the scope of *ācāra.*

There are four basic elements that help us to distinguish ritual from ordinary behavior; they are (1) formality, (2) pattern, (3) sequence, and (4) repetition. When a particular behavior exhibits these four characteristics, we can identify it as a ritual. Religious acts are most obviously identified as rituals, but it is important to realize that human behavior in a nonreligious context can also be ritualistic. The significance of rituals can be well understood by observing animal life. Animals are known to behave ritualistically when they court or fight. Such ritualized behavior prevents the animals from reacting excessively to the conflicting situations.

Laboratory experiments have shown that rituals help to engage and focus attention, heightening discrimination, enhancing multidimensional generalization, and improving associative learning (Fernald 2002). Rituals work by capturing attention to the signal elements of the ritual that can evoke a response from the receiver. Exaggeration of ordinary traits and behaviors is a characteristic feature of rituals. The exaggeration of ordinary behavior makes a ritual very formal. This formality helps to activate regions of the brain like reticular formation, basal ganglia, and amygdala. This helps to gain control of emotions and focus the attention. This helps the individual to respond to situations with awareness. Even in the animal species, ritualistic behavior has been found to play a crucial role in successful adaptation by bringing about alterations in neurophysiology (Hauser and Konishi 1999; Searcy and Nowicki 2005). Rituals help in regulating behavior.

6.3 Well-Being

We can thus see that ritual and dharma are intricately interconnected. Ritual helps to establish dharma which in turn creates *saukhya* or well-being. *Saukhya* refers to quality of life and must be distinguished from standard of living. The term for standard of living is *kṣema*. It has been shown that sense of well-being, as much as it can be measured, does not necessarily increase correspondingly with the comfort that results from increasing income. As a result, standard of living should not be taken as a critical measure of well-being. Well-being is not just happiness, which can be momentary. Well-being is a state of inner satisfaction that is more stable. In a state of complete well-being, one is satisfied with one's state of health, personal relationships, safety, standard of life, achievements in life, social relationships, and identity, as well as prospects for the future (see Chap. 9 in this volume). In Āyurveda, these aspects of well-being have been considered under three categories: security of life (*praṇaiṣaṇā*), standard of living (*dhanaiṣaṇā*), and secure future (*paralokaiṣaṇā*) (Yadavji 1992).

> There are three pursuits to be engaged in which are security of life, pursuit of wealth and the afterlife (Ćaraka Saṃhitā, Sūtra Sthāna, 9, 3 in Yadavji 1992)

The well-being of the people of a nation can be measured in terms of these three parameters: secure living conditions, high living standards, and good prospects for the future.

In Āyurveda, well-being is defined at both the individual and social levels. A life that leads to individual well-being is known as *sukha āyu*, and the life that promotes social well-being is known as *hitam āyu* (Yadavji 1992). Pursuit of individual well-being can run into conflict with social well-being. It is a challenging task to discover a way of life that will be conducive to both individual and social well-being. The solution is dharma.

Dharma helps one to establish a life that leads to personal and social well-being.

6.4 Dharma

The connection between rituals and well-being revolves on the fulcrum of dharma. It is difficult to define dharma and therefore what is the right *karma*. The ancient texts point out that even the most enlightened people in society are unable to define what is dharma and what is not.[1]

[1] http://sanskritdocuments.org/sites/completenarayaneeyam/new-fffsansMainIndex.htm. Accessed in June 2012.

> Even the sages are confused when it comes to defining what is *karma* and what is *akarma* (Bhagavad Gītā, 4, 16 in Ramsukhdas 1995)

One has to observe the actions of people who act with a clear conscience to understand what is dharma.

> The principle of dharma is hidden and elusive, the way of dharma is the life of the great people itself (Mahābhārata, Vana Parva, 313, 117)[2]

In a broad sense, however, dharma is action that confirms to the basic unity of the universe. To acknowledge the unity of the universe, it is needed to recognize the relationships between different entities that will lead to harmony and sustainability on a long-term basis. From this perspective, it has been said that the essence of dharma is to put oneself in the position of the other in any given situation. Sage *Vyāsa* appeals in the *Mahābhārata* to hear and understand that the essence of dharma is to not do unto others what one would not do unto oneself.

> Listen and understand that in the ultimate analysis dharma means not doing unto others what you would not do unto yourself (Mahabhārata – Udyoga Parva, 15, 17)

In another context in the *Mahābhārata*, Sage *Vyāsa* is seen lamenting that his advice is not being heeded by the people. He says that one obtains lasting wealth and pleasure only by adhering to dharma, yet people refrain from complying with it

> I am literally crying with both my arms lifted upwards but no one heeds my words. Both wealth and pleasure are obtained by adhering to dharma, yet why is it that people do not follow *dharma*? (Mahabhārata – Svargarohaṇika Parva 6)

In the social context, *dharma* is that which resolves the conflict between the pursuit of personal and social well-being. It would be interesting to analyze how some of the most common and simple social rituals aim to establish *dharma* and thereby well-being.

6.5 The Ritual of Salutation

The ritual of salutation in the Indian tradition can be taken as a simple illustration to drive the point home. The salutation that is exchanged when two people meet is known as *namaskāra* in the Indian tradition. The *namaskāra* is a highly ritualized form of salutation or greeting. It is different from a casual greeting because of its ritualistic character. Many of the rituals are actually exaggerations of good conduct in society. *Namaskāra* literally means to bow down. It is performed by bringing the two palms of the hands together close to the chest in front of the region of the heart and also slightly bowing the head forward at the same time. It is a noncontact form of salutation unlike shaking hands, embracing, or kissing. It is, in fact, the gesture

[2] http://www.holybooks.com/mahabharata-all-volumes-in-12-pdf-files/. Accessed in June 2012.

of praying that is prevalent in many cultures of the world. *Namaskāra* is a ritualistic way of preparing for a social interaction. The bringing together of the palms of the two hands is to greet the other person in a prayerful mood. This symbolizes the union of the heart of the two individuals before initiation of interactions. It is done to invoke the mood of cooperation and mutual goodwill to ensure that personal well-being does not conflict social well-being. The fact that there is no body contact in *namaskāra* is an acknowledgement of physical differences between individuals. *Namaskāra* is an acknowledgement of spiritual unity while accepting physical, mental, and cultural differences.

There is an interesting narrative in the *Bhāgavata Purāṇa* that throws light on the significance of *namaskāra* as a ritual for salutation. This narrative is also thought provoking for pointing out the futility of rituals when they become rigid and fixed. The context of the narrative is the encounter between *Śiva* and *Dakṣa*. To cut a long story short, *Dakṣa* had to accommodate *Śiva* as his son-in-law when *Sati*, his lovely daughter, offered herself in marriage to Śiva. During a gathering, *Śiva* fails to salute *Dakṣa*, who takes offense and curses him. The sequel of events that followed culminates in the self immolation of *Sati*. During a conversation in the midst of all this drama, *Śiva* explains to *Sati* the meaning and significance of the salutation ritual

> As regards exchange of formalities in the shape of rising from one's seat and advancing to meet a friend, respectful behavior and salutation etc., O slender waisted lady, it is properly done only by the wise, who do all this mentally with respect to the Supreme Person dwelling in every heart, and not to him who regards the body as his own self. It is the absolutely pure mind which is termed as *Vāsudeva*, because it is there that Supreme Consciousness is realized in its unmasked glory. It is in the shrine of such a mind that I offer *namaskāra* or salutation (Cited in Śrīmad Bhāgavata Purāṇa, by Anonymous 1989)

Śiva declines from performing salutation, the very *namaskāra* ritual, which had become established by tradition as a mandatory custom in social interactions. *Śiva*, the God himself, becomes a nonconformist. This narrative illustrates the point that rituals have relevance so long as they serve the purpose of upholding dharma. A ritual is broken when it fails to fulfill its purpose. Thus, the making and breaking of rituals constitute a dynamic process to establish dharma in social life in the cultural traditions of India.

Anthropologists have suggested that rituals in many societies serve the purpose of resolving conflicts of reciprocal relationships between individual, small group, community, and society. The analysis of the Bedouin practice of *Bisha*, the ordeal of fire, by Al-Krenawi and Graham demonstrates that the ritual reflects the social order and reinforces conformity to collective values (Al-Krenawi and Graham 1999). O'Gorman with the study of social norms put forth the argument that confirming to group identity and social norms affects individual and social success (O'Gorman et al. 2008).

We can propose that social rituals help in executing social norms and patterns of behavior, which in turn help groups and communities to be more successful by collective action. These actions help in establishing collective identity (Hermanowicz and Morgan 1999).

6.6 Marriage, Animal Sacrifice, and Wine Ceremony

The *Bhāgavata Purāṇa* also discusses at length on the ritualization of marriage, meat eating, and drinking liquor. This *Purāṇa* points out that the inclination towards sex, meat, and alcohol is natural and people indulge and get infatuated by these sensory pleasures without any provocation (cited in Srimad Bhagavata Purana by Anonymous 1989).

> People are prone to indulge in sex, meat and alcohol without any provocation, whatsoever (Śrīmad Bhāgavata Purāṇa, 11, 5, 11 by Anonymous 1989)

In order to curb these tendencies, the institution of marriage, the ritual of animal sacrifice, and the wine ceremony have been established (cited in Śrīmad Bhāgavata Purāṇa by Anonymous 1989).

> Marriage, animal sacrifice and wine ceremony are means to curb and regulate the instinct for indulgence in sex, meat and alcohol (Śrīmad Bhāgavata Purāṇa, 11, 5, 11 by Anonymous 1989)

The institution of marriage has been ritualized to such an extent that the bonding between the couple is made sacrosanct. And in the process, the sexual activities of the individuals become confined within the boundaries of married life. The *Bhāgavata Purāṇa* is explicit when it says that one of the purposes of marriage is to regulate the sexual life of people. Unbridled sexual propensities can lead to violent and criminal behavior in society and can also disrupt relationships and harmony in society. From the point of view of health and well-being, Āyurveda imposes several restrictions and regulations on sexual activity. Regulated sex is considered as one of the three pillars of life and is an important component of lifestyle management.

If unchecked, the urge to eat meat can lead to widespread slaughter and cruelty to animals. Traditions of health, like Āyurveda, acknowledge the utility of meat not only in maintaining health but also in treatment of diseases. And the issue of whether eating meat is against dharma is taken up for discussion in the medical texts. Eating meat for the sake of sensual gratification is considered to be against dharma (Harisastri 2002).

> The killing of birds and animals to protect one's body which is an instrument for *yajna* or sacrifice is not against *dharma*. On the other hand, killing animals for the sake of pleasure and enjoyment is *adharma* (Aruṇadatta on Aṣṭāṅga Hṛdaya Saṃhitā, Sūtra Sthāna, 1, 1 in Harisastri 2002)

On the other hand, eating meat for medical reasons, to protect one's body, is considered as *dharma*. The ritual of animal sacrifice was constituted to regulate the killing of animals and overindulgence in eating meat. To eat meat, one should kill the animal by performing a ritual, which imposed a restriction on widespread killing of animals. The ancient texts also point out that one form of life is food for another, thus acknowledging the food chain and food web in nature. The idea is that there is no need to provoke people to eat meat; the tendency is instinctual. Animal sacrifice was a check on cruelty to animals and not a sanction for animal slaughter. The *Mṛgapakṣiśāstra*, a medieval text on Zoology, narrates the change in the mindset of a King who goes hunting to the forest. On reaching the outskirts of the forest, the King is suddenly overwhelmed by the biodiversity and the richness of wild life that he encounters. Remorseful of his hunting expedition, the King returns to the palace and commissions the composing of a book that describes the different species of animals and birds to create awareness of and respect for animal life (Nalini Sadhale 2008).

The worship of the cow is another related ritual that seeks to protect animal life. The cow has been given the status of motherhood, and this is affirmed by the enactment of rituals to ensure that cows are cared for like mothers. The simple fact that cows provide milk for humans is sufficient reason to confer it with the status of a mother. The purpose of the ritualistic worship is to establish an emotional bond between cows and humans that would prevent exploitation and ensure care and protection. Snake worship and the concept of the sacred grove are likewise based on the principles of protection of animal life and eco-conservation. Snakes were worshipped in the sacred groves, and these rituals symbolized the allocation of habitat for snakes that was kept undisturbed by human interference. The sacred groves were also biodiversity hotspots, where rare and endangered animal and plant species were preserved. Such rituals are related to well-being at spiritual and ecological levels.

In one of the texts of Āyurveda, it is prescribed that one must look at even an ant or insect as oneself (Harisastri 2002).

> One must look upon even an ant as one's own self (Aṣṭāṅga Hṛdaya Saṃhitā, Sūtra Sthāna, 2, 23 in Harisastri 2002)

While this is an attitude to be developed, the ritual of *kolam*, which consists of decorating the front of one's homes with patterns and designs made of rice flour, is a practical way to provide food for ants and other lower forms of life.

Consumption of alcohol has great potential to turn into a social evil. And it is not easy to keep people within restraints in this matter. The ritual of drinking wine was established with the goal of regulating the use of liquor. As in the case of eating meat, the wine ceremony is not a sanction for indulgence in liquor but rather a regulation imposed by ritualizing it. Āyurveda is again quite explicit when it comes to describing the medicinal properties of alcohol. Ayurvedic texts include a subsection on liquors and wines in the chapter that lists food items. Āyurveda also suggests that liquor inebriates in three stages and that the first stage of inebriation provides health benefits. Specific liquors are recommended as appetizers and digestives. Fermented products that have alcohol content are part of the most common dosage forms for medicines used in Āyurveda. Āyurveda warns that liquor has very little medical value in tropical climate but can be helpful in a cold environment (Harisastri 2002).

> In the summer season, one must not consume alcohol or drink it after diluting it with plenty of water (Aṣṭāṅga Hṛdaya Saṃhitā, Sūtra Sthāna, 3, 29 in Harisastri 2002)

But the fact that liquor can cloud one's intelligence and provoke actions that cause social disharmony is reason enough to keep it at a distance from oneself (Harisastri 2002).

> The use of liquor is prohibited for the simple reason that it clouds one's intelligence (Aṣṭāṅga Hṛdaya Saṃhitā, Nidāna Sthana, 6, 10 in Harisastri 2002)

Moreover, liquor has poisonous and toxic properties that can wreak havoc on one's physical health (Harisastri 2002).

> Alcohol is antagonistic to the inner vitality known as ojas (Aṣṭāṅga Hṛdaya Saṃhitā, Sūtra Sthāna, 6, 1 in Harisastri 2002)

Ayurvedic texts have not absolutely contraindicated the consumption of alcohol, while *madyātisakti* or excessive consumption is prohibited (Harisastri 2002).

The brewing, selling, buying, and distribution on a mass scale have been prohibited outrightly (Harisastri 2002).

Marriage, animal sacrifice, and wine ceremony are examples of three rituals originated in a religious context but aimed to regulate social behavior by tempering instincts that could potentially lead to social disharmony and conflicts. We can thus see that one purpose of rituals was to temper the instincts of the human mind. Sensual propensities are compared with the power of horses. Just as one controls the horses by alternatively releasing and pulling the reins, the sensual instincts can be controlled only by indulging and restraining at the same time. This is exactly the mechanism through which these three rituals are intended to work. The mind that has tempered its instincts is composed and can participate in social interactions by confirming to collective values.

Ironically enough, the rituals of animal sacrifice and the wine ceremony have been abused to such an extreme that the very purpose for which they were conceived has been defeated. The *Bhāgavata Purāṇa* itself talks about the violation of these rituals and condemns the people who indulge in these rituals without understanding their significance (cited in Śrīmad Bhāgavata Purāṇa by Anonymous 1989).

> Ignorant people slaughter animals in the name of religious sacrifice and take false sanction from the scriptures. They violate their own self and the Lord in other life forms and live a wretched life. (Śrīmad Bhāgavata Purāṇa, 11, 5, 14 by Anonymous 1989)

6.7 Impact of Rituals on Different Aspects of Well-Being

Rituals impact well-being at different levels. In the Indian tradition, the main goal of rituals has been to establish dharma, which is more than just social order. Rituals also have preservation of life (*āyu*), promotion of health (*ārogya*), creating prosperity (*aiśvarya*), social recognition (*yaśas*), and secure sense of future (*śāśvata loka*) as their goals. These are all different dimensions of well-being. Rituals aim to establish both personal and social well-being (see Fig. 6.2).

There are many rituals that aim to promote health (Bradley 2008). A temple ritual in Kerala distributes medicated buttermilk as the blessings (*prasāda*) of the deity. This buttermilk improves digestion, metabolism, and immunity of the body. Ritualization in a temple setting facilitated the distribution of this medicated drink to significantly large number of people in the society. Another ritual, followed also in Kerala, is to consume medicated rice gruel during the rainy season. The ingredients of this medicated food help to strengthen the body and ward off diseases that manifest during the

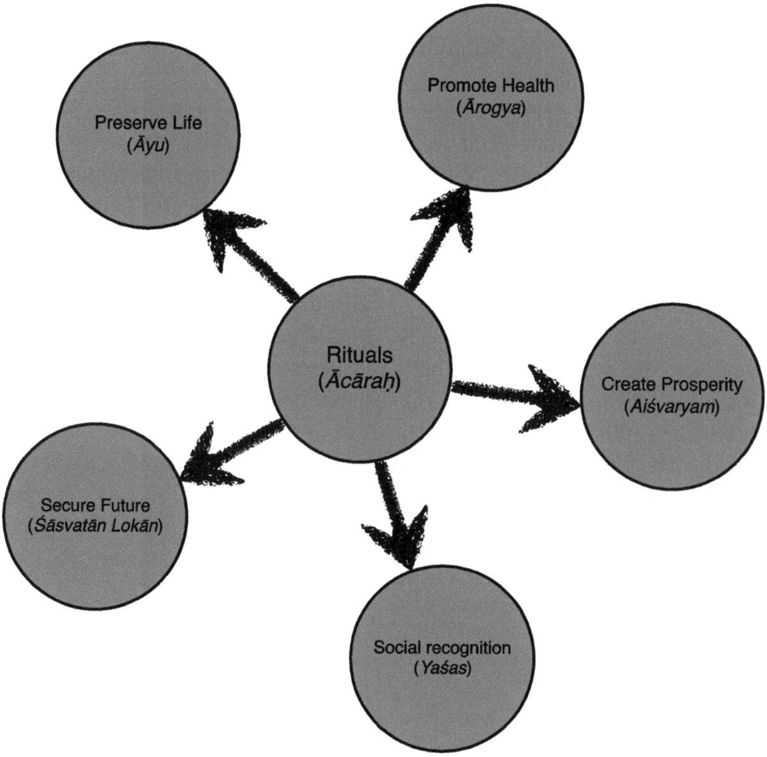

Fig. 6.2 The impact of rituals on well-being. The eight aspects of well-being that are experienced by adherence to ritualized behavior are depicted in this diagram

rainy season. Once again, the ritualization of this practice makes a large section of the society to follow and practice it. The practice of ritual fasting on prescribed days helps to bring self-control, to moderate the diet habits, and also to tone up the digestive system. Many of the temple rituals have been formulated with a view to inculcate healthy lifestyle. These rituals require one to wake up in the wee hours of the morning, take long walks in the temple, bathe in the pond, and get fresh air from the trees and plants growing in the vicinity.

There are rituals that celebrate prosperity, and some of these coincide with harvest festivals. Such festivals kindle social cooperation and distribution of resources in the society (Rappaport 1999). The *Onam* festival in Kerala is associated with a variety of rituals and beliefs that aims to promote equality and prosperity in the society. The *Onam* festival is based on the belief that King *Mahābali*, the ancient ruler of Kerala, will visit the homes of his subjects once in a year. The reign of King *Mahābali* represented prosperity and well-being par excellence. People adhered to dharma and were blessed with all-round well-being. The rituals performed during *Onam* festival highlight the values of equality, sharing of resources, and harmony in social life by adherence to dharma. Temples have also served as centers for equitable redistribution of wealth. The temple is the altar to offer possessions that one is most attached to. In the act of offering, the donor chants – "this is not mine, this is not mine."

The temple becomes a resource pool to store and redistribute excess wealth accumulated by individuals for social welfare. The recent discovery of unimaginable riches stored at the *Sri Padmanabha Swamy* Temple in Thiruvananthapuram, Kerala, testifies how effective temples were in collecting excess wealth from society. It is estimated that the value of the riches of this temple is about US$23.94 billion, which would make it the richest temple in the world. However, over a period of time, the system of redistribution of the hoarded wealth declined and became dysfunctional. Offering of free food on a daily basis (*annadānaṃ*) and distribution of clothes (*vastradānaṃ*) are part of temple rituals to ensure that the basic needs of people in society are met. The Ayurvedic texts insist that one should not be concerned with one's well-being alone (*naikaḥ sukhī*). Most of the temple rituals, called *yajñas*, have fair distribution of wealth and resources as its basis. The *Bhagavad Gīta*, for instance, explains that the concept of *yajña* is inbuilt with life. *Yajña* or cooperation, sharing, and sustainable use of resources is the wish-fulfilling cow of human kind (Ramsukhdas 1995).

> The creator infused the principle of self sacrifice into the entire creation and proclaimed that all living beings may procreate and flourish by relying upon this principle as their wish fulfilling cow – (Bhagavad Gītā 3, 10 in Ramsukhdas 1995)

6.8 The Sixteen Civilizing Rituals

The sixteen civilizing rituals (*ṣoḍaśa saṃskārās*) are yet another example of rituals that promote well-being in human life. These include sixteen rituals that are performed from birth to death, which start from the prenatal period. The *samskaras* help family and friends to get together and create social bonding, which forms the basis for a peaceful life. They also create an identity to the individual and help in establishing links and relationships with the society at large. The civilizing rituals represent important stages in life. They alert individuals and society to prepare and come to terms with the key milestones in the cycle of birth and death and take measures to preserve life, promote health, and create prosperity. Of the sixteen rituals, three are performed before birth, six in the stage of infancy, three in childhood, three in adulthood, and one at the time of death. As it can be seen, the majority of the rituals pertain to childhood, and by early adult life, all but the death ritual is completed. This points to the fact that the foundation for a good life has to be laid during childhood and that the effort has to start before conception itself. These rituals helped the people in the society to consciously participate in the psychosocial evolution of life (see Chap. 3 in this volume).

The three rituals that are performed before birth are *garbhādhāna* (planned pregnancy), *pumsavana* (exercising choice in the sex of the progeny), and *sīmantonnayana* (ceremonial parting of the hair of the pregnant woman). A child should be conceived by choice rather than chance. Attempt was made to beget a male child by using medications in the early stage of pregnancy in families that did not have a male child for many generations. The *sīmantonnayana* ritual aims to protect the pregnant woman in the most critical stage of her pregnancy. It helps to sensitize everyone in the family to provide extra care and attention for the expectant mother.

The rituals that are performed in the stage of infancy aim to give identity and protection to the child and help in giving social recognition to the child. The *jātakarma* is done immediately after birth and consists of medications that aim to enhance the immunity of the child. The *nāmakaraṇa*, or naming ceremony, gives identity to the child. The first outing of the child, when it is exposed to the external world and society, is known as *niṣkramaṇa*. The child is given solid food for the first time by performing the *annaprāśana* ritual. The child's head is shaved in the third or fifth year leaving a tuft of hair at the back, and this ritual is known as *cūḍākaraṇa*. It is believed that this ritual helps the child to eliminate memories of past lives; in other words, it symbolizes the beginning of a new life. It is also believed that shaving the head helps to stimulate healthy hair growth. This is then followed by the *karṇavedhana* ritual, which is the piercing of the earlobes. This is best done when the child is still in its infancy and the earlobes are soft and easy to pierce. One obvious reason for piercing the ears is to decorate it with earrings, but there is also a belief that it helps to stimulate the vital point (*marma*) at the tip of the earlobe, providing some health benefits.

Three rituals are performed in the stage of childhood. When the child is about 5 years old, it is initiated into the process of education. The child becomes literate by getting introduced to the letters of the alphabet. This ritual is known as *vidyāraṃbha*. When the child is 8 years old, it is taken to the teacher for initiation into formal schooling. This is symbolized by the wearing of the sacred thread called *upanayana*. *Upanayana* means to bring close, and here it means to take the child to the vicinity of the teacher. The ritual that marks the study of the scriptures is known as *praiṣārtha*. This consists of two smaller rituals called *upakarma* and *upasarjana* performed at the beginning and end of the academic sessions. These rituals aim to enforce systematic education for the child.

The rituals of early adulthood mark the entry of the child into adult life. In males, at the age of 16, the hair is removed ceremoniously. This is known as *keśānta*. This marks a period of transition in the child's life and the development of the adult personality. In case of the girl child, the ritual performed is known as *ṛtuśuddhi*, indicating menarche marking the transition of the girl into a woman.

At the end of formal education, the ritual called *samāvartana* is performed. This is very similar to the graduation ceremony and marks the end of the celibate life of studentship. The next ritual is *vivāha* or marriage, and after this is completed, man and woman become husband and wife and enter the stage of the householder (*gṛhasthāśrama*).

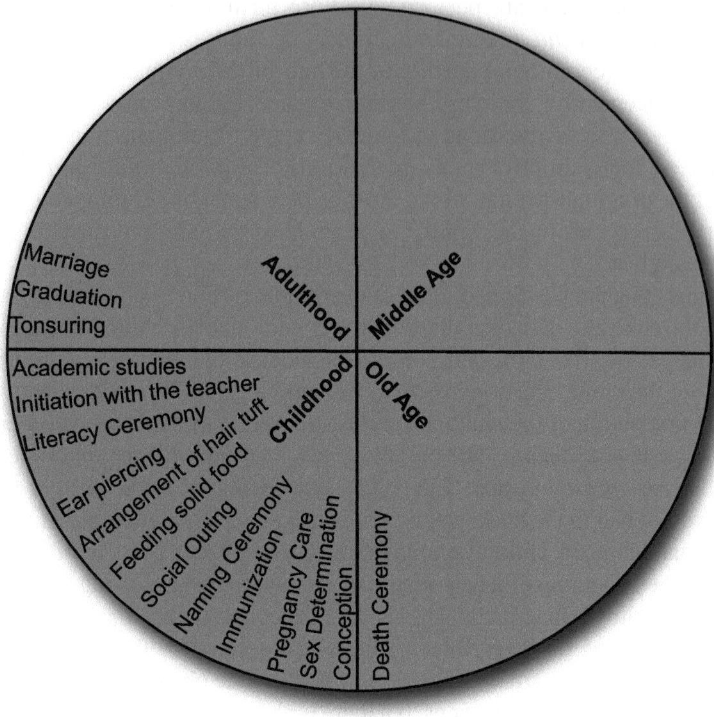

Fig. 6.3 Fifteen of the sixteen civilizing rituals (*saṃskāras*) are completed by early adulthood implying that the foundation for well-being has to be laid in early part of life. This diagram reveals that ritualized behavior is more important in the younger formative stages of life

Fifteen of the sixteen rituals are completed with marriage, and the remaining ritual is *antyeṣṭi* or the death rites. Death is tackled in a ritualistic manner, and this helps the members of the family and society to manage the psychological trauma caused by the separation and to come to terms with the inevitable consequence of life.

The fifteen civilizing rituals pertain to important phases in human life, where the correct attitude and decisions can make the difference between success and failure in life. Some of the rituals represent phases in life, where the individual goes through emotional or intellectual or social transformations. The message is that if one takes the proper steps from prenatal life to marriage, then one can live one's life to its full potential and face death with a sense of fulfillment. Thus, the sixteen ritual program aims to make best use of the early part of human life to lay the foundation for a life that will be established in all-round well-being (see Fig. 6.3).

There are different opinions on the number of the *saṃskāra* or civilizing rituals. The number ranges from 12 to 42 in various ancient texts. It is likely that these rituals have evolved and might have been modified in the course of time. But the underlying principles have remained unchanged. The rituals have been rediscovered and redefined to save them from the rigidity that they acquire in course of time. And they serve as the roadmap to prepare and come to terms with the changing phases in the journey of life. So much so that one is established in a state of inner and outer well-being.

There are rituals that are based on the principle of using the power of intention of the human mind to influence the course of life events of the individual as well as of nature. It is beyond the scope of this chapter to enter into a discussion on these specialized rituals.

6.9 Transcending the Bondage of Rituals

Rituals will fail in their purpose if they do not succeed in achieving all the dimensions of well-being. Spiritual well-being is an important goal of dharma and thereby of rituals. True awareness of dharma is synonymous with spiritual well-being, as both represent awareness of the unity of the universe. What then to say if rituals come in the way of spiritual well-being? By spiritual well-being is understood the expansion of awareness from self-centeredness to universe centeredness (see Chap. 9 in this volume).

When spiritual well-being is achieved, one perceives oneself in the universe and the universe in oneself (Yadavji 1992).

> True intelligence perceives the world in oneself and oneself in the world (Ćaraka Saṃhitā, Śārīra Sthāna, 5, 7 in Yadavji 1992)

When the inner significance of rituals are not understood, rituals become mere external enactments and devoid of purpose. The ancient texts have pointed out this danger and strongly criticized people who perform and misrepresent rituals for selfish gains or without any purpose. The *Bhagavad Gītā* makes mockery of people who indulge in rituals only for the sake of prosperity and individual well-being. It points out that spiritual well-being is never attained by those who do not understand the real implications of the rituals they perform (Ramsukhdas 1995).

> The intelligence of those people will not attain equilibrium, who preach in flowery words that there is nothing beyond the Vedas and who are lost in the pursuit of enjoyment and wealth (Bhagavad Gītā, 2, 42–43 in Ramsukhdas 1995).

The *Bhagavad Gīta* outrightly rejects obsessive adherence to the *Vedic* rituals and condemns such people as fanatic supporters of *Veda* (*vedavādaratāh*). The same text also says that the *Veda* deals with the three *guṇa* of nature, purity, delusion, and ignorance and that one must transcend the three *guṇa* to attain spiritual well-being (Ramsukhdas 1995).

> The subject matter of *Veda* is within the scope of the three material *guṇa*. O! *Arjuna*! Go beyond the *triguṇa* (Bhagavad Gītā, 2, 45 in Ramsukhdas 1995).

When spiritual well-being is achieved, one is ever established in the awareness of *dharma*. Rituals become superfluous in this state. The *Nārada Bhakti Sūtra* brings forth this idea very clearly by saying that a person who has attained spiritual well-being forsakes rituals and the *Veda* (Ravisankar 2003).

> A spiritually enlightened person discards all rituals and even the *Veda* – (Nārada Bhakti Sūtra, 3, 15–16 in Ravisankar 2003).

Ādi Śankara points out that those who get carried away by the external pomp of rituals fail to grow spiritually. People may quote the scriptures, make sacrifices to the gods, perform actions, and pay homage to the deities, but there is no liberation without recognizing the unity of the self with the universe, not even in the lifetime of a hundred *Brahma* (countless millions of years).

> Let them quote from the scriptures, offer sacrifices to the gods, perform many actions, and pray to deities. Liberation will not be attained without realising the oneness of the individual and cosmic self. (Vivekacūḍāmaṇi of Ādi Śaṅkara 1, 6 in Madhavananda 1982)

Spiritual awareness comes with tempering of the mind. The mind is tempered by adherence to *dharma*. Rituals help in establishing *dharma*, they create the circumstances for the psycho-spiritual evolution of the mind, which has to be initiated and completed consciously. In modern times, Rabindranath Tagore has pointed out the meaninglessness of rituals performed without sense of purpose. The lines from his thought-provoking poem "Go not to the temple" are worth quoting here:

> Go not to the temple to put flowers upon the feet of God, First fill your own house with the Fragrance of love…, Go not to the temple to light lamps before the altar of God, First remove the darkness of sin from your heart… Go not to the temple to bow down your head in prayer, First learn to bow in humility before your fellowmen…Go not to the temple to pray on bended knees, First bend down to lift someone who is down-trodden. …Go not to the temple to ask for forgiveness for your sins, first forgive from your heart those who have sinned against you[3]

That purity and innocence of the mind that is the true basis of temple worship is highlighted by an anecdotal account from the life of *Narāṇan* the lunatic. *Nārāṇan* was a vagabond-exhibiting eccentric behavior, but many of his actions, seemingly conveyed profound messages, had a reformative influence on society. As he was wandering around the village one day, he came in front of a temple, where the priests were struggling to consecrate the deity. Elaborate rituals were being performed, but the idol was not getting positioned in place. *Nārāṇan* was much amused by what he saw and, without heeding the protests of the onlookers, took hold of the idol in his hand, spat the betel quid that he was chewing on the altar, and placed the idol over it saying "Now, you stay here in place." The legend goes that much to the surprise of everyone, the idol became stable and well positioned on the altar. The moral of this story is that rituals are insignificant and meaningless when purity of the heart is attained.

Rituals are practices that groom behavior and align the human mind with the highest *dharma*: the appreciation of the unity of the universe. Rituals have relevance until the sense of dharma is fully awakened, after which they become redundant.

[3]http://mptbc.nic.in/books/class11/enggt11/ch1.pdf

Rituals guide and regulate action in individuals who have not cultivated awareness of *dharma*. On the other hand, rituals performed out of context do not lead to awakening of the sense of dharma and in such cases become counterproductive and needs to be discarded.

6.10 Conclusions

In the Indian cultural tradition, rituals have been associated with well-being. This association is made explicit in the medical traditions of Āyurveda. Rituals establish well-being by enforcing *dharma*, or the universal order. *Dharma* includes unity among members of society, ethical values, sustainability of nature, and human endeavors and stands for all actions that lead to social and individual well-being (Sosis 2004; Rappaport 1999). Rituals also aim to inculcate control over senses and emotions by enforcing discipline. This is achieved by ritualizing good conduct by exaggerating behavior and formalizing them into repetitive and sequential patterns. Rituals help to establish well-being in terms of preservation of life, enhancement of health, creation of wealth, social identity, and sense of security for future life, by creating unity in minds of individuals and grooming the emotions. Rituals lose their power and significance when they become rigid and fixed. It then becomes necessary to break, rediscover, and redefine them. The validity and utility of a ritual lies in its power to establish dharma and thereby social and individual well-being. When rituals are performed with awareness and conscious effort, it becomes a powerful tool for self-transformation and well-being.

References

Al-Krenawi, A., & Graham, J. R. (1999). Conflict resolution through a traditional ritual among the Bedouin Arabs of the Negev. *Ethnology, 38*, 163–174.

Anonymous. (1989). *Srimad Bhagavata Purana*. Gorakhpur: Gita Press.

Anonymous. (2010). *Vishnusahasranama*. Gorakhpur: Gita Press.

Bradley, T. (2008). Puja as one dimension of a sensitive, relational approach to community health care provision. *Journal of Religion and Health, 47*, 504–515.

Fernald, R. (2002). Social regulation of the brain: Status, sex and size. In D. Pfaff, A. Arnold, A. Etgen, S. Fahrback, & R. Rubin (Eds.), *Hormones, brain and behavior* (pp. 435–444). New York: Academic.

Harisastri, P. V. (Ed.). (2002). *Ashtanga Hridayam*. Varanasi: Chaukhambha Orientalia.

Hauser, M. D., & Konishi, M. (Eds.). (1999). *The design of animal communication*. Cambridge, MA: The MIT Press.

Hermanowicz, J. C., & Morgan, H. P. (1999). Ritualizing the routine: Collective identity affirmation. *Sociological Forum, 14*(2), 197–214.

Madhavananda, S. (1982). *Vivekacudamani of Sankaracarya*. Kolkata: Advaita Ashrama.

Nalini Sadhale, Y. L. N. (2008). *Mrigapakshishastra*. Secunderabad: Asian-Agri-History Foundation.

O'Gorman, R., Wilson, D. S., & Millerd, R. R. (2008). An evolved cognitive bias for social norms. *Evolution and Human Behavior, 29*, 71–78.

Ramsukhdas, S. (1995). *Srimad Bhagavad Gita*. Gorakhpur: Gita Press.
Rappaport, R. A. (1999). *Ritual and religion in the making of humanity*. Cambridge: University Press United Kingdom.
Ravisankar, S. (2003). *Narada Bhakti Sutra*. Bengaluru: Vyakti Vikasa Kendra.
Searcy, W. A., & Nowicki, S. (2005). *The evolution of animal communication: Reliability and deception in signaling systems*. Princeton: Princeton University Press.
Sosis, R. (2004). The adaptive value of religious ritual. *American Scientist, 92*(March–April), 166–172.
Yadavji, T. (Ed.). (1992). *Ćaraka Samhita*. New Delhi: Munshilal Manoharlal Publishers Pvt. Ltd.

Chapter 7
Health and Well-being in Indian Local Health Traditions

Unnikrishnan Payyappallimana

7.1 Introduction

A description about health and well-being in Indian scenario is promising when contextualized in a biocultural[1] and an ecosystem perspective. An ecosystem approach reiterates the innate, dynamic relationship between nature and humankind and hence biological and cultural diversity as well as communities' belief systems and perceptions of health and well-being. Such a consideration is especially important for local health traditions which are ecosystem and community specific and health and well-being concepts and practices are highly embedded in local worldviews and value systems. This exemplifies multiple benefits derived from ecosystems towards health and well-being through various natural resources such as food, medicine and shelter to recreational, cultural and aesthetic values through ecological landscapes including sacred healing sites (Millennium Ecosystem Assessment 2005[2]). For instance, India represents around 7 % (numbering around 17,500) of all identified flowering species of the world. As high as

[1]Biocultural diversity denotes an inherent linkage between a wide array of life forms and their ecosystems and environments on the one hand and the range of human expressions. In totality this diversity encompasses genes, species, ecosystems, landscapes and seascapes to worldviews, belief systems, knowledge, morals, values, norms, languages, rules, artistic expressions, artefacts and institutions of a region that have generally been passed on through an intergenerational transmission process and shared by a group. They mutually and constantly evolve in response to a changing environment or world order (Haverkort 2006).

[2]Millennium Ecosystem Assessment (2005) Biodiversity and Well-being: Synthesis Report, Island Press.

U. Payyappallimana (✉)
United Nations University-Institute of Advanced Studies, Yokohama, Japan

Institute for Āyurveda and Integrative Medicine, Bangalore, Karnataka, India
e-mail: unnipm@gmail.com

A. Morandi and A.N. Narayanan Nambi (eds.), *An Integrated View of Health and Well-being*, Cross-Cultural Advancements in Positive Psychology 5, DOI 10.1007/978-94-007-6689-1_7,

9,000 plants are used in the traditional communities of the country for various purposes such as food and medicine (AICRPE 1992–1998), of which around 8,000 are used for medicine (Shankar and Unnikrishnan 2004). This typifies the deep human-nature relationship and the wealth of knowledge in local health traditions.

For a clearer appreciation of this relationship, one may look at the classification in classical Sanskrit literature of Indian cultural life into three categories: *aranya* (forest related), *gramya* (rural) and *nagarya* (urban). Historically, while this classification may have corresponded to different levels of sophistication in lifestyles, demographic patterns as well as knowledge codification, today it represents a more complex yet nearly corresponding picture. Even as we recognize that such a distinction may be obscure as most communities are in rapid transition due to various socioeconomic factors, it gives a broad framework for analysis on the influence of nature in the sociocultural life and its impact on health and wellness.

According to 2001[3] census of India, out of total population of 1,027 million, about 285 million live in urban areas (in over 5,100 towns and 380 cities) and 742 million live in rural areas. As per the census, India has a tribal population comprising of 8.2 % of total population, who live inside or in close proximity to the forests. Also known as *adivasis*, they are categorized on the basis of geographical isolation, distinct culture, language and traditions by the Indian Constitution. Even with relatively rapid urbanization in the country, many of the traditional communities have retained their lifestyles, community life, knowledge and related value systems. Some groups follow subsistence agriculture and land holdings if existing are small. They continue to closely relate with the forests for several of their needs such as food, fuel and medicine and earn livelihoods through traditional occupations including selling minor forest produce like fruits, honey, tubers and medicinal plants. The second group, which is considered here as *gramya*, is involved in agriculture and related occupations and consists of roughly 50–60 % of Indian population. This represents rural economies comprising of communities from buffer areas of forests, villages to shanty towns or suburban areas. The third group is those who live in urban areas, representing around 28 % of the population.

The point to note is that roughly over half of the Indian population continues to associate with natural landscapes and ecosystems and uphold traditional lifestyles in their daily lives and occupations. Consequently, the health and well-being perceptions of a large section of the population are around this relationship. The range of social life represents a complex milieu with regard to status or perceptions of health and well-being among rural communities. This varies vastly in terms of determinants, access, availability, affordability and quality of health care. They also continue to be guided to a considerable extent by access, belief systems and their capabilities in traditional health practices.

[3] See India census data: http://www.censusindia.gov.in/Census_Data_2001/India_at_glance/rural.aspx

7.2 Characteristics of Local Health Traditions

In India, in terms of knowledge or usage of traditional medicine, a clear geographical or societal demarcation of folk as well as codified knowledge traditions is impossible. Traditional lifestyles either deriving from codified knowledge traditions or from the folk cultural practices are followed beyond geographical or class boundaries. Such practices may relate to textual, inherited, incorporated or experiential knowledge and skills (Sujatha 2007).

However, the phrase *local health tradition* here denotes the geographical and ecosystem-specific practices, beliefs, customs, rituals related to health, nutrition or broader well-being passed on from one generation to another mostly in oral transmission. It is to be noted that folk knowledge practices also have been documented and exist in the form of regional and vernacular literature, while a considerable part of codified traditions is part of family traditions and not necessarily from classical texts. Terms like folk, little traditions (as opposed to great) and indigenous knowledge are used interchangeably to indicate such practices though any of these terms may not fully represent the intricacies of this tradition. These traditional practices represented by knowledgeable households, folk healers and other community knowledge holders are mostly non-institutional and non-codified. It includes what is popularly known as grandmothers' remedies, the household knowledge about primary health care, different health food recipes, seasonal health regimens and health customs, rituals, etc. This also covers over a million community-based health workers belonging to various specialties such as bone setting, specialized in jaundice, paralytic conditions, children's diseases, eye diseases, poison healers, spiritual healers and birth attendants. They range from specialized diagnostic techniques to management methods related to preventive, curative and promotive aspects of health. Healing is mostly not a full-time profession for such practitioners, and they may be a farmer, barber, shopkeeper, blacksmith, teacher or even priest or a monk. One of the reasons for the widespread nature of this tradition even today is the low sustenance cost and a noncommercial nature. Such practitioners have no formal recognition of education but continue to serve in communities due to social legitimacy and community support (Shankar and Unnikrishnan 2004).

A recent study by Lohokare and Davar (2010) on traditional mental health practitioners in Maharashtra says that 'a nuanced approach that appreciates the centrality of healing in the larger socio-cultural context of well-being and community life is critical. Indigenous healing systems are mistakenly seen in a homogenous light, completely obscuring their internal variations that exist between different systems'. The study points out how such local traditions positively contribute to the transcendental and existential aspects of health and well-being which are context specific and beyond universalization, an important feature of local health traditions. Shared explanatory frameworks, healing practices including rituals, physical healing environment and so on become central in such a context. Despite variations in social structures (such as caste or religion), the concept of ecology, body, health and disease is more or less uniform among people, resulting in the medical lore of a particular group. Such a 'medical lore' which is endured and refined through generations has its 'coherence' and 'epistemological autonomy' and is quite different from 'lay knowledge', and this is not an amateur version of classical, codified knowledge. Such knowledge is mainly deriving from communities' perceptions of bodies and the outside environment (Sujatha 2007).

7.3 Co-evolution and Sharing Among Knowledge Traditions

Whereas there are two distinct knowledge streams such as the local health traditions (*loka*) and the codified knowledge systems (*śāstra,* which are codified and institutionalized), they share many of the concepts and practices in common and have a complementary relationship. These are reflected in several of the cardinal concepts and essential principles of these knowledge traditions. For instance, the *loka-puruṣa* or the microcosm and macrocosm relationship as mentioned in Āyurveda is also a central dimension in the local health traditions. Similarly underlying theoretical aspects such as *pañcamahā bhūta* theory (theory of composition of matter) and *tridoṣa* theory (theory of causation of health and disease) are also shared in various ways by these systems. Though such classifications may not be obvious in folk expressions, this can be deduced from the usage of several technical terms such as *uṣṇa, sīta, guru, laghu, vāta, pitta and kapha* by the folk knowledge carriers (Balasubramanian 2003, 2006). There is also a huge overlap of the medicinal resources used by these knowledge streams. Some of the other aspects shared are the focus on systemic understanding of health and diseases; multicausality approach; a circular method of cause-effect reasoning; subjective, qualitative, individualized and personalized management; preventive focus; attribution of importance to physician's wisdom; and so on. Another unique shared feature is that knowledge generation is mostly through subtle observations and experiences within the context, i.e. an individual or the nature (Payyappallimana 2010). Such interactions and exchanges are core elements in health knowledge production in the subcontinent. Such continuum and complementarities are found also between *Siddha* medicine and current folk perceptions of food and nutrition, health, illnesses and their management in Tamilnadu. Often the outcomes of these exchanges are more complex and layered than a mere dichotomy such as 'folk' or 'classical' systems (Sujatha 2007).

There are two dominant views related to the generation and codification of knowledge in Indian health traditions. First, according to Ayurvedic classical literature, the preceptor (*brahma*) 'remembered' the knowledge of life which was passed on to the disciple *prajāpati* who in turn successively transferred this to Aswini kumaras, then to Indra and his disciples who codified the knowledge in present form. The second view is that local, oral health knowledge perceptions and practices (*prākṛit*) have been collated, theorized and codified into textual traditions such as Āyurveda. In such a view, forests and related communities are bestowed with abundant knowledge and resources. Both positions receive equal attention right from the time of earliest codified medical text, i.e. *Ćaraka* Saṃhitā. A passage in *Ćaraka* Saṃhitā says:

> shepherds, cowherds, and those living in the forest are knowledgeable about medicinal materials both by name and form (Ćaraka Saṃhitā, Sūtra Sthāna, 1, 120 in Sharma and Dash 2001)

or in other words, wilderness is a rich repository of health knowledge. According to *Dhanvantari Nighantu* (200–1000 AD), those who live in proximity to the natural environments have a clear idea about the measurements (*pramāṇa*), colour (*varṇa*), physical characters (*ākriti*) and the specific reproductive characteristics (*jātiliñga*) of each plant, pointing to the fact that such traditions were consulted extensively. Whereas there have been some changes in the relationship between these two streams after institutionalization of the codified traditions in the last 100 years and their formal recognition in the health system, there still exist active exchanges between these traditions. The following section will dwell briefly on the relationship between the two and knowledge codification. This assumes importance in appreciating how health and well-being perceptions and practices have evolved in communities.

According to Indian philosophical traditions, any knowledge or practice is conceived at three levels of existence of a being. They are first, at the level of physical existence relating to the practical aspects (*vyavahāra* – practical applications), second at the mental level relating to the methodological/scientific aspects (*śāstra* – dos and don'ts) and third at the level of inner self (*ātman*) where the individual becomes one with the object (*tattva* – essential principle) or the essential nature of it. In other words *tattva* is the essential truth/principle relating to a particular practice, symbol, ritual, etc., and this is an understanding at the level of *ātman* (self). *Śāstra* relates to the do's and don'ts which is linked to *manas and buddhi* (mind and intellect) and *vyavahāra* is related to *indriyas* (*jñanendriya* and *karmendriya* – tools of knowledge and action). These three levels also correspond to the three frequent questions that arise constantly in us such as 'why', 'how' and 'what', respectively. To put it in a different way, through a repeated practical experience (*vyavahāra*), one recognizes the *sukha* (pleasure) and the *dukha* (pain) of an experience. This experience gives the individual a framework (the do's and don'ts) of relating to that experience or similar experiences in their temporal and spatial dimensions (*śāstra*). Through such continuous experiences and reflection, one internalizes the *tattva* (essential nature) of the experience. It is also indicated in classical texts of Āyurveda that *tattva* reflects itself in a clear or uncomplicated mind (Payyappalli and Hariramamurthi 2011).

If one looks at the dynamic nature of traditional knowledge, it can be seen that the 'practical aspects' are known to most members in a community; in other words it is a shared community knowledge and varies or changes vastly based on the needs of time and geographical context – while the 'methodological aspects' which are more specialized also vary, though to a lesser degree, according to time and context. But the third level which is the wisdom of 'essential nature' remains unchanged. This describes the process on how practical or local knowledge experiences are codified and theorized to apply in different spatial and temporal contexts as in the classical literature; at the same time, how codified knowledge continuously verifies and guides practical actions. It is explicit that the codification process need not necessarily be textual. This also reiterates how the codified and non-codified knowledge have had a mutually nourishing relationship and have been co-evolving.

7.4 Local Health Traditions, Ecosystems and Health and Well-being

Defining health in a broader context of well-being is challenging due to the encompassing nature of these terms and is often criticized as too idealistic. It is also argued that such a definition aims at conceptualizing health as a positive attribute to be achieved through universal health coverage of modern health care while neglecting the understanding of health as a socioculturally constructed attribute. The much acclaimed definition of WHO considers health as a 'state of complete physical, mental and social well-being and not merely the absence of disease or infirmity' (WHO 1948). In a similar optimistic tone, this view is also shared by the local health cultures which take into account mental, social, spiritual, physical and ecological dimensions of health and well-being. In local communities it emerges from the idea of relationship between the being and nature or the macro- and microcosm. A fundamental concept is of equilibrium of these dimensions within an individual, individual and community, the two together with the environment and the larger universal space. Any breach in this nexus leads to disease (Bodeker 2009), which is a shared view of health in Indian traditions. In yet another view of Indian healing traditions, the absence of incapacitating disease, good psychological functioning, effective conduct of personal and social life and feeling of ethical and spiritual well-being are defining elements of good health (Kakar 1982).

The intricate linkages of health and well-being with the nature and sociocultural factors are reflected in these definitions. There is increasing realization that nature and ecosystems are the bedrock of services that lead to health and well-being as they provide health and nutritional resources, spiritual and recreational spaces, inspiration and a learning and identity space for communities in proximity. This indicates the centrality of the health of ecosystems to ensure health of individuals and communities. In the contemporary view, health of the ecosystem correlates to morbidity patterns, life expectancy and quality of life and the sustenance of a productive engagement of the communities with the environment. Specifically, regulation of pests and disease-causing pathogens, availability of good-quality water and well-functioning ecosystem services are essential to ensure well-being. It is to be noted that human health and well-being are dependent not just on the direct ecosystem services derived from the proximate environment.

Various cultural expressions such as festivals, rituals, customs and value systems in traditional communities reinforce this relationship with nature ensuring an inspirational milieu. This also extends to a realm of knowledge generation in local healing traditions. A healer derives inspiration for healing methods as well as medicinal resources from the landscape with which he or she interacts. This is shared by tribal healers in most other parts of the country. For instance, in Wayanad region of Kerala state, healers mention that their healing prowess and approaches are revealed through dreams or visions. They also say that the drugs reveal themselves to (and often communicate with) them (Suneetha 2004). A healer in Gadchiroli in Maharashtra, during a field visit, indicated that the constant interactions with the natural environment give them a sense of what is good for health and what is poison. This is a sense of heightened consciousness of the healer within the biocultural mosaic. A child who grows up in such an environment instinctively learns about processing and the use of medicinal resources for a variety of ailments. Following her study in Baiga region of Central India, Sarangapani (2003) says, 'In Baghmara village, for instance, virtually all the adults have a fairly extensive knowledge of the trees and plants in the forest, and varying degrees of knowledge about the medicinal properties of various plants. Children, both boys and girls, from the age of about 5 or 6 years can identify several of the more common medicinal plants around the village. On a few occasions they mentioned what it was used to treat; typically stomach ailments. By the age of about 8 or 9 years, the scope of the child's environment and knowledge both widen quite dramatically. On some of our visits together to the forest, they named over 60 plants with medicinal properties, and many more that bore fruits that could be eaten or were useful. They stopped their list out of consideration for me because I could no longer keep track…'. Proximity to a biodiversity rich natural surrounding unsurprisingly provides a vast knowledge of medicinal plants and other resources. This continues to be a unique aspect of local health traditions as against the institutionally qualified traditional medicine physicians who today hardly recognize wild resources or appreciate the broader social and environmental determinants of health and well-being.

Within this broad backdrop, an attempt is made as follows to illustrate some of the distinctive features of local health traditions with regard to health and well-being. These categories include underlying principles, beliefs, determinants, drivers or means of health and well-being in local communities.

7.4.1 Microcosm and Macrocosm

A shared perspective across communities is the inherent relationship between the 'outside' and 'inside' worlds. Whereas this is refined in Āyurveda and other codified systems of medicine in terms of '*loka*' (macrocosm) and '*puruṣa*' (microcosm), traces of this principle form an underlying basis for all local traditions. This is apparent in the tenets of balancing the 'internal' and 'external' environments. This then leads to identifying similarities and differences in *rūpa* (form), *guṇa* (quality) and *karma* (action) of materials and methods which are central to recognizing drug resources or health management principles. For example, in terms of medicinal resources, body parts such as hair, skin, blood and flesh or their qualities or functions are compared with external materials and in turn identified as medicines for a condition in the corresponding body part or function. Use of *haridra* (turmeric) for jaundice, *lakṣa* and *manjiṣta* (lac, *Rubia cordifolia* and other similar plants that are *red* in colour) for haemorrhage or goat's milk for respiratory disorders, in folk knowledge traditions exemplify this principle. Another interesting and illustrative example is the usage of *Garudakodi* (an Aristolochia species), literally translated as eagle twiner for *sarpaputtru* (a viral condition literally translated as snake hills) and articulated in a shared myth across communities, which exemplifies such local taxonomies originating from this understanding of the nexus of inside and outside worlds. Likewise, external manifestations such as flow, transformation or degeneration in the form of metaphors are applied as diagnostic or therapeutic categories which also represent the inherent link.

7.4.2 Spiritual Dimension and 'Beyond Self' Pursuits

Extending from the above, a human being is considered a miniature of the infinite external world, as against an anthropocentric view. Therefore, this reflects the need for a being to be integrated well with the larger whole, forming the basis of a spiritual aspiration and pursuit. Divinity to the external world is attributed through symbolic representations, earmarking sacred resources, spaces and time. This is also echoed in the way a healer derives knowledge from his/her environment through dreams or intuition where there is a thinning of line between the nature and the divine.

Likewise deep reverence to ancestry is an abiding tenet in traditional cultures. This includes predecessors within the family, community and teachers. Such ancestors are invested with a guardian role of supporting, protecting and guiding various activities of individual and communities. Hence, there is immense value placed on appeasing ancestral spirits to ensure own well-being. The presence of a higher power is also ascribed to the healing powers of a healer. Some healers are considered to have been gifted with special healing powers that is referred to as 'the power of the hand' or *Kaippunyam* (see Box 7.1). Healers themselves consider that they work as instruments of God, further affirming that the knowledge they possess is the 'word of God' (Suneetha 2004). The concept of the impact of positive and negative actions of a being on the larger whole is also central. For instance, the practice of offering prayers and conducting rituals before cutting a plant for medicinal purposes, as seen in many traditional communities in India, is illustrative – the consequences to the life form harvested is duly acknowledged.

Spirituality is also expressed in the material resources. For instance, some disease conditions such as chronic skin ailments are believed to be caused by both physical and spiritual factors, and it is common to find healers advise patients to make specific offerings to the snake gods before starting the treatment. Offerings are also made in the case of ailments such as chicken pox to the Goddess Kali (Hafeel et al. 2003). The Gond community in Vishakhapatnam in Andhra Pradesh believes in existence of an array of divine beings and ancestral spiritual forces that dwell in houses, community spaces, fields, burial grounds and forest areas. It is believed that they can help or harm and are beyond the control of human beings. It is also believed that they help and protect in situations of danger. In order to appease the spirits, so as to protect them from evil influences, the communities conduct rites and rituals. This is also followed before any important event at home such as a house construction, land preparation, tree felling or marriage proposals. There is the belief

Box 7.1 Healing Hands of Shimoga

Near Shimoga, southern India, Mr. Narayana Murthy is a living example of how a local healer is effectively contributing to community health. For the past two decades, he has been serving the people on 2 days (Thursday and Sunday) every week. These days are considered as Siddhi varas – days which give good effect. The healer and his family are strong believers of God and do the daily rituals as per community rules. The blessing of the community deity (Lakshmi narasimha) is an important factor which influences the patient's well-being and efficacy of the medicine given.

Healer Murthy treats the patients without any charge. The family's source of income is agriculture. Patients are allowed to put money in the metal box with small opening, without any condition, and this amount is later used to meet the expenses of their community temple. Most cases that come to him are diagnosed cancer of different kinds (70 % according to him) and people often consider this place as a final place of hope. Some patients carry laboratory reports of clinical diagnosis and hospital discharge summaries. His 'one-day' medication for the urinary calculi and medicines for heart blocks are a well-known remedy in Karnataka and adjacent states.

According to the patients, their belief in the good heart and genuine mind of the healer is essential in the healing. As they state: 'we only want the medicine from his hands'. The Murthy family has established 30 acres of land with naturally grown medicinal plants and tree species. Healer Murthy views the plant as a living and a life-giving organism and a specific ritual is needed when collecting the required plant part. This ritual is a pradakshina, encircling the divine body of the tree. He prays for the effect of the medicine and asks permission of the tree to take its part with medicinal properties. He says that this ritual bestows the effect of medicine. The ritual is also a sincere prayer for the benefit of each patient who comes to him for treatment (Adapted from Hafeel et al. 2003).

that Mother Nature guards and protects them, as they are believed to be the children of nature. The sacredness is attributed to trees, grains, animals, hills, forests, streams, mountains and caves that are worshiped through rituals, ceremonies, festivals and fairs. Such knowledge, belief systems and worldview find expression in agro-ecological traditions, arts, songs and other symbolic representations, practices linked to well-being (Shankar 2003).

Individual well-being is achieved within the broader realm of community well-being. While individual welfare is not ignored, it is dovetailed with the broader well-being of the community of which the individual is a member. This gives rise to a non-self-centred approach that provides for individual needs, while exacting sacrifices for the overall welfare of the group or the community. Further, the concept of rebirth and time as a cyclic phenomenon also plays down the finality of death, sometimes even celebrating the occasion as a passage of rite. Therefore, among some communities, well-being of current, past and future lives are believed to have equal significance.

7.4.3 Natural Resources and Health

This covers aspects such as medicinal resources, nutritional resources and the recreational aspects related to biocultural diversity. Diversity of foods, their availability and processing methods during different seasons contribute to nutritional and health security of communities. This perception of health is ingrained in local cuisines and exemplified in the use of an array of spices and adjuvants in traditional cooking methods specific to different agro-climatic regions. In a study in communities of coastal Tamilnadu, Sujatha (2007) mentions, 'the body is seen as being constituted by food which is the vehicle by which the external ecology is internalized'. Communities use regularly four to five millets such as finger millet, pearl millet, kodo millet and little millet along with several different sources of vegetables. Communities assert that diversity in food is important as it facilitates balancing effects of deficiencies in a uniform diet, acclimatizes the body to diverse elements in the habitat and thus contributes to a healthy body.

The diverse and continued use of medicinal plants, minerals, metals and animal products/parts among some communities is astounding. For example, a study conducted in the hamlet of Bommiampathy in the Attappady region of Kerala reveals that around 500 medicinal plant species are used within the hamlet (Unnikrishnan 2009). It is noteworthy that each of such local communities uses about three times as many resources as documented in Āyurveda. Local traditions swiftly incorporate new additions to the repertoire of medicinal resources or knowledge which allows the traditions to be in a state of dynamic refinement. There is a belief among communities that plants available in local area will be more effective for a population residing in a particular location. This has resonance in the classical Ayurvedic understanding. Āyurveda adds that resources from place of origin will be effective even if one has migrated to a new locale.

Festivals, ceremonies and rituals which continue to be practised in communities have a direct bearing on well-being. There is growing body of research on the impact of festivals on physical and mental health and in reinforcing identities, resilience and capacity at individual level as well as at community level (Phipps and Slater 2010). In India though many festivals and rituals have religious functions, they also have strong links with local healing traditions. For instance, there are festivals or rituals such as for marking the harvest season and prosperity (i.e. *Pongal*), related to procreation (i.e. *Thiruvathira*) and rejuvenation (i.e. *Karkidaka* regimen in Kerala) to mention a few from South India. The direct health impacts are reflected in the various medicinal and nutritional resources used in these festivities. For example, the Ugadi festival marks the New Year in the states of Karnataka, Maharashtra, Andhra Pradesh and Goa. It symbolizes the differing life experiences of sadness, happiness, anger, fear, disgust and surprise which need to be greeted in a balanced state and equanimity. A medicated mixture among several other traditional dishes consumed during the occasion is believed to represent these varied experiences and consists of materials like neem buds and flowers (bitterness, signifying sadness), jaggery and ripe banana pieces (sweetness, signifying happiness), pepper (pungent, signifying anger), salt (signifying fear), tamarind juice (sour, signifying disgust) and unripe mango (astringent, signifying surprise).[4] The impact of such festivals and rituals, both direct and indirect, on health and well-being has not been well documented and studied in Indian context.

7.4.4 *'Health Is from Within'*

Health is an attribute of self-reliance and control of own life of an individual. Though rapidly changing, there is a strong belief among older generation that health cannot be created merely with external means such as medicines. In a recent reconnaissance survey conducted in Kerala among elderly (75 years is the average life expectancy in the state), the respondents mentioned that health is dependent on a disciplined lifestyle, a life in moderation, promoting aspects of self-healing in the body, regular exercise and having a composed approach. This also alludes to the notion that health is a balance of internal and external elements mentioned earlier. Based on a study in Thirupathur taluk area in coastal Tamilnadu, Sujatha (2007) says that the communities in the region believe that disease is part of the body and no one is free from it as its proneness or manifestation is linked to the constitution. Owing to constitutional variations, different parts of processes are likely to malfunction. Multiple causes are reasoned for a manifestation; however, the prime source is within the body and the 'quality of blood' which is linked primarily to the diet and lifestyle. If these two are taken care of, an external agent or pathogen cannot breach the body.

7.4.5 *Carriers of Health and Well-being*

In an analysis of health-seeking behaviour of communities, Kleinman[5] identifies three arenas of care: home, nonprofessional and professional. He further adds that at the home level, beliefs, choices, relationships and interaction with others, engagements with institutions and health products play a critical role and that 75 % (750 of every 1,000 illness episodes) never get outside of family sector. At the level of the

---

[4] See http://www.manavata.org/Events/ugadi.htm

[5] See Arthur Kleinman, National Institute of Health lecture, 2002: http://videocast.nih.gov/Summary.asp?File=10463

nonprofessionalized folk sector, local healers and lay therapists play a vital role, while in the professional sector, hospitals, clinics of biomedical medicine, Chinese medicine or Ayurvedic medicine are important.

In the Indian context, it is true that most of the common ailments especially in the rural milieu are managed at household level or within the community. Most household women know local remedies for common primary health conditions. At the second level, there exists variety of informal knowledge carriers such as local healers, diviners, magic or religious practitioners engaged in community health. An important agency of intergenerational transfer is through oral processes such as proverbs, songs, stories involving health, healing resources and management approaches, which reinforce ideas of health and well-being. Healers also pass on their knowledge to next generation by choosing them based on qualities that are valued in tradition, such as patience, faith, courage and keenness for healing (Payyappalli 2010).

7.5 Changes and Challenges

The concepts related to health and well-being in this context, as mentioned earlier, are characterized by a dynamic nature. Due to rapid socioeconomic transition, these practices are in a state of flux. The emergence of a mainstream market for health products and services, more accessible than before; changes to the social relations within a community to a more individualistic frame with resultant consequences to resource ownership and use (such as land, waters); changes to extant percepts of health and well-being among the community members; and increasing outmigration away from their ecosystems into more prospective territories are some of the challenges. There is high erosion in the local traditional knowledge and practices both in household as well as more specialized healers' level. This is evidenced from the fact that average age of a healer is over 50 years and there are not many successors. At the household level, the reducing usage of local medicines can be attributed to erosion of knowledge, inconvenience and improved access to and availability of conventional medicines. Such erosion has a considerable impact on health and well-being especially in areas where access to health care is a problem. Codification of such traditions through documentation methods has risen in recent times through various policy and implementation programs.

7.6 Conclusion

The central role of traditional medicine, conservation of ecosystems and natural resources in achieving better human health and well-being, is being increasingly recognized in multilateral policy discussions. There is also a renewed interest in primary health care, with the revival of this approach by the World Health Organization in 2008. Several multilateral conventions and resolutions uphold the relevance of biodiversity and traditional knowledge in health and well-being of the people especially in regions with poor access to health care, yet rich in natural resources.[6]

This chapter attempted to highlight this relevance of informal health knowledge streams of India in this context. The discussion was purposively positioned on the contemporary relevance of local health traditions (than a historical or ethnographic narration) with regard to community health and well-being. While a clear demarcation of folk and classical knowledge or their geographical patterns of usage is not possible, it can be assumed that roughly over 50 % of the population continues to have strong association between their sociocultural landscapes and natural environments and thus actively engage with traditional medical knowledge systems for their primary health and nutritional needs. This nexus extends over diverse aspects such as medicinal resources, food and nutritional resources, protection from epidemics or spiritual and recreational aspects which are central to health and well-being. There are several challenges such as rapid changes in sociocultural life, erosion of knowledge practices, emerging market forces, demographic changes, migration, changing health and well-being perceptions in communities among others. Keeping these in mind, effective policy interventions are essential to strengthening such practices. This indeed calls for a participatory approach to health care in which individuals and communities become active and self-reliant stakeholders in actualization of health and well-being.

References

AICRPE (All India Coordinated Project on Ethnobiology). (1992–1998). *Final technical report*. New Delhi: Ministry of Environment and Forests, Government of India.

Balasubramanian, A. V. (2003). Knowledge and belief systems in the Indian subcontinent. In B. Haverkort, K. Van Hooft, & W. Hiemstra (Eds.), *Ancient roots new shoots – Endogenous development in practice*. London: Zed Books.

Balasubramanian, A. V. (2006). Is there an Indian way of doing science? In A. V. Balasubramanian & T. D. Nirmala Devi (Eds.), *Traditional knowledge systems of India and Sri Lanka*. Chennai: Compas Series Worldviews and Sciences, CIKS.

Bodeker, G. (2009). In G. C. Cook & A. I. Zumla (Eds.), *Manson's tropical diseases* (22nd ed., pp. 35–45). London: Saunders Elsevier.

[6]For instance, in the conceptual framework for poverty and ecosystem of United Nations Environment Program (UNEP) and International Institute of Sustainable Development (IISD), the ability to use traditional medicine and 'continue using natural elements found in ecosystems for traditional cultural and spiritual practices' are two of the 10 resources of well-being (UNEP & IISD 2004). Similarly in the United Nations Committee on Economic, Social and Cultural Rights resolution of 2000, Article 34 on the right to the highest attainable standard of health, states' obligations to respect include '[…] to refrain from prohibiting or impeding traditional preventive care, healing practices and medicines'. Convention on Biological Diversity (CBD) has called for increased synergies between CBD and WHO for improving linkages of ecosystems, biodiversity and community health.

Hafeel, A., Suma, T. S., Unnikrishnan, P. M., & Shankar, D. (2003). Reviving local health traditions. In B. Haverkort, K. Van Hooft, & W. Hiemstra (Eds.), *Ancient roots new shoots – Endogenous development in practice*. London: Zed Books.

Haverkort, B. (2006). Dialogues within and between different sciences: Issues and strategies from endogenous perspective. In B. Haverkort & C. Reijntjes (Eds.), *Moving worldviews – Reshaping sciences, policies and practices for endogenous sustainable development* (pp. 345–362). Leusden: ETC/Compas.

Kakar, S. (1982). *Shamans, mystics and doctors: A psychological inquiry into India and its healing traditions*. London: Unwin Paperbacks.

Lohokare, M., & Davar, B. V. (2010). The community role of indigenous healers in health providers. In K. Sheikh & A. George (Eds.), *India – On the frontlines of change* (pp. 161–181). New Delhi: Routledge.

Millennium Ecosystem Assessment. (2005). *Biodiversity and well-being: Synthesis report*. Washington, DC: Island Press.

Payyappalli, U. (2010). Knowledge and practitioners: Is there a promotional bias? In S. Subramanian & B. Pisupati (Eds.), *Traditional knowledge in policy and practice: Approaches to development and human well-being* (pp. 194–207). Tokyo: UNU Press.

Payyappalli, U., & Hariramamurthi, G. (2011). Local health practitioners in India – Resilience, revitalization and reintegration, medicine, state and society In V Sujatha & L. Abraham (Eds.), *Indigenous medicine and medical pluralism in contemporary India*. New Delhi: Orient Blackswan (in press).

Payyappallimana, U. (2010). Role of traditional medicine in primary health care: An overview of perspectives and challenges. *Yokohama Journal of Social Sciences, 14*(6), 57–77.

Phipps, P., & Slater, L. (2010). *Indigenous cultural festivals: Evaluating impact on community health and well-being*. Melbourne: Globalization Research Centre, RMIT University.

Sarangapani, P. M. (2003). Indigenising curriculum: Questions posed by Baiga Vidya. *Comparative Education, 39*(2), 199–209. Special Number (27): Indigenous education: New possibilities, ongoing constraints.

Shankar, G. (2003). Building on tribal resources. In B. Haverkort, K. Van Hooft, & W. Hiemstra (Eds.), *Ancient roots new shoots – Endogenous development in practice*. London: Zed Books.

Shankar, D., & Unnikrishnan, P. M. (2004). *Challenging the Indian medical heritage*. New Delhi: Foundation Books.

Sharma, R. K., & Dash, B. (Translators). (2001). *Ćaraka Saṃhitā*. Varanasi: Chaukhamba Sanskrit Series Office.

Sujatha, V. (2007). Pluralism in Indian medicine: Medical lore as a genre of medical knowledge. *Contributions to Indian Sociology, 41*(2), 169–202.

Suneetha, M. S. (2004). *Economic valuation of medicinal plants in the context of convention on biodiversity and intellectual property rights regulation*. Department of Agricultural Economics, University of Agricultural Sciences, Bangalore, India (Unpublished).

UNEP & IISD. (2004). *Human well-being, poverty and ecosystem services: Exploring the links, UNEP, IISD report, 2004*. http://www.unpei.org/PDF/economics_exploring_the_links.pdf

Unnikrishnan, E. (2009, March 22). Āyurvedathinu Ayussundo. *Mathrubhumi* (in Malayalam).

World Health Organization. (1948). *Constitution of the WHO*. http://apps.who.int/gb/bd/PDF/bd47/EN/constitution-en.pdf. Accessed on 26 April 2013.

Part III
Bridging the Worlds

Chapter 8
Quantum Logic in Āyurveda

Rama Jayasundar

8.1 Healthcare: Emerging Trend

Western medicine, which is striving to provide professional healthcare system with the aim of eradicating diseases, has undergone an explosion of knowledge leading to diagnostic and therapeutic breakthroughs. Yet, the disease burden has not reduced and the overall results in terms of complete cure without side effects have left much to be desired (Dean 2005; Gandhi et al. 2003; Lazarou et al. 1998; Moore et al. 1998). A number of diseases previously under control are no longer manageable with the currently available medicines. For example, new strains of drug-resistant bacteria have developed, which defy treatment with conventional antibiotics (Goossens et al. 2005; Hawkey and Jones 2009). In addition, factors such as altered lifestyle and environmental conditions are also contributing to new health threats. Diseases now defy state-of-the-art diagnosis and treatments (Avenell et al. 2004; Illich 2003; Mackenbach 2006; Shahri and Hagemann 2011).

It is becoming apparent that despite specialised knowledge and use of sophisticated technologies, modern medicine seems unable to handle the mushrooming of diseases underscoring the need for a relook at alternative approaches to medicine. Moreover, with an increasingly chemicals-weary population turning to alternative systems, a pluralistic and integrated approach to healthcare is emerging world over (Bishop and Lewith 2010; Wade et al. 2008). Even in Western countries at the forefront of modern medical research, there is growing interest in alternative systems of treatment (Kemper et al. 2008; Morandi et al. 2011; Xue et al. 2007). This inevitably brings into focus one of the longest unbroken healthcare system in the world, i.e. Āyurveda, indigenous to Indian subcontinent. As Western medical science contemplates alternative approaches, it is pertinent to understand Āyurveda, whose

R. Jayasundar (✉)
Department of NMR, All India Institute of Medical Sciences, New Delhi, India
e-mail: ramajayasundar@hotmail.com

A. Morandi and A.N. Narayanan Nambi (eds.), *An Integrated View of Health and Well-being*, Cross-Cultural Advancements in Positive Psychology 5, DOI 10.1007/978-94-007-6689-1_8,

concepts and approaches to health and diseases are at variance with that of Western medicine (Jayasundar 2009, 2012a) but resonate with some of the concepts of quantum physics applicable to the macroscopic world. This chapter explores points of contact between Āyurveda and quantum physics, in particular quantum reality and worldview. It also gives a bird's-eye view of the two streams of medicine – the currently prevalent classical physics-based reductionistic Western medicine and the vedic sciences-based holistic Āyurveda.

8.2 Classical Worldview and Western Medical Science

Physics has been very influential in shaping the development of biology and medicine. It has contributed tremendously to the advancement of medical diagnostics such as ultrasound, Computerised Tomography (CT) and Magnetic Resonance Imaging (MRI) and therapeutics like nuclear medicine and radiotherapy. From x-rays to laser, applications of physics have been successfully translated into medical technologies (Davidovits 2007; Kane 2009). While these contributions of physics are well appreciated, very little is understood about the impact of its worldview in medicine. That it has influenced medicine in a way more than one can appreciate is much less known. Before we explore how worldviews have shaped medicine, it is imperative to know the development and specific viewpoints on health and disease of both the Western and Āyurveda systems, both of which are outlined in brevity in the following sections.

8.2.1 Classical Worldview

The classical/Newtonian physics deals with macroscopic objects and the forces governing them. Its laws formulated in terms of physically describable variables have been extended with tremendous success from atoms to terrestrial bodies. Physics came to be known as deterministic physics since the entire physical universe from the smallest to the largest was seen to be bound by these laws and the concept of physical determinism (Burtt 1952; Butterfield 1997). A worldview based on this had emerged by nineteenth century, which considered the world as being made up of building blocks of atoms. This Newtonian worldview considered everything from human body to universe as a machine composed of separate interacting material particles/objects behaving in accordance with the physical laws. According to this worldview, even nature could be reduced to fundamental entities of matter. This viewpoint became the platform from which everything, including biology and medicine, was viewed and understood. Consequently, human body also came to be considered as being made up of building blocks of atoms and molecules. More importantly, the focus has been on the physical aspects (as in classical physics) with elements of the mental realm completely left out. Consequently, body and mind also came to be viewed as two entirely separate entities in Western medicine.

8.2.2 Western Medical Science

Hippocrates, the father of Western medicine, brought in for the first time the concept of logical rather than supernatural explanations for illness. Since dissection of human cadavers was forbidden on religious grounds then, he relied primarily on logic and tangible evidence to understand health and disease. He considered the latter a result of imbalance among the four humours (blood, black bile, yellow bile and phlegm), each of which was also associated with a personality type. Centuries later, Galen (130–201 AD), a Greek philosopher and physician, extrapolated human anatomy from that of pigs, which was considered most similar to humans. The Hippocratic-Galenic theories on the body-mind-personality relationship and views on anatomy dominated Western medicine for the next 1500 years (Conrad et al. 1995; Nutton 2004).

The dissection of human cadavers of executed criminals by Vesalius in 1539, following a landmark judgement, corrected the mistaken notions of human anatomy proposed by Galen and marked a historical milestone in Western medicine. However, developments such as the discovery of blood circulation by William Harvey in 1628 began an era of viewing human body as an assemblage of organs supplied with energy/fuel by blood. The use of microscope to view cells by Robert Hooke in 1664 marked yet another stage of development in Western medicine. Slowly, symptoms till then considered to be natural physiological responses to disease began to be viewed as pathologic consequences and the body-mind-personality connection fundamental to Galenic medicine was also discarded (Conrad et al. 1995; Nutton 2004; Ventura 2000). The concept of linear and singular causality for diseases, however, started with Morgagni's work connecting aetiology of diseases to specific anatomical locations (Ventura 2000). This marked the beginning of pathological anatomy, which focuses on a single, dominant factor considered responsible for a pathology and uses it for targeting treatment.

Impact of Classical Worldview on Western Medicine: Reductionism

While the above-mentioned developments in the field of medicine set the stage for understanding human body from a predominantly mechanical perspective, advances in physics played a crucial role in catalysing and developing them further. The Newtonian mechanistic worldview considering the world as being made up of fundamental units of matter as building blocks became the platform for the reductionistic approach in medicine. Reductionism as a systematic method to understand the world was proposed by Descartes, who suggested the world was clock-like and could be understood by reducing it to parts and studying the individual components (Cottingham et al. 1988; Haldane and Ross 1911). This concept of breaking down of a complex system into smaller parts and studying them separately has been a very successful approach in biology for studies ranging from understanding the working of cells to the unravelling of human genome (Keller 2000; Morange 2001).

The reductionist model is hierarchical, with atom in the lowest level forming the basic building block. Atoms make molecules, which in turn form cells and then tissues. A group of tissues working together form an organ and a group of organs referred as an organ system perform a major function. The human body is understood in terms of various systems such as skeletal, circulatory, and reproductive. Disease is understood and treated at the lowest level of the structural hierarchy, i.e. at molecular level (Conrad et al. 1995). Treatment is corrective and generally involves bringing deviated parameters within normal range. For example, diabetes is marked by hyperglycaemia, making this parameter the focus of conventional diabetes management – the treatment aims directly at correcting the deviated glucose level. Corrective treatment is based largely on control or suppression of symptoms by manipulating the body's chemistry with drugs. Methodological reductionism, thus, pervades clinical medicine from diagnosis to therapeutics (Morange 2001; van Regenmortel and Hull 2002).

Caveats in Reductionism and Changing Perceptions

The reductionistic approach, though very effective in providing significant information on biology and disease processes, has not been able to translate its success from bench to bedside for delivering complete cure without side effects. Much of this is attributed to the limitations of reductionism, which focuses on the identified molecular target but excludes the rest of the system (Beresford 2010; van Regenmortel and Hull 2002). There is increasing realisation that this compartmentalised approach underestimates the complexities of biological systems. For example, this approach views brain in terms of wired circuits and chemical processes with even consciousness and mental states reduced to chemical reactions (Bickle 2003; Ito 2006; Miller 2011). The classical idea of matter and linear causality of diseases may not be compatible with the complex nature of various processes involved in brain because not only are the synapses non-linearly connected but there is also causal effect by conscious experience (Libet 2003). Although one cannot ignore the strengths of the reductionist approach, the question whether it is still valid in clinical medicine as once thought is being increasingly asked by biologists (Joyner 2011). There is now a slowly changing perception that the structural/chemical constituents in an organism are not in isolation but are in dynamic relationships, which decide the overall functioning of not only the cells and organs but the entire organism. There is also a growing appreciation that no part can be understood outside of the whole to which it belongs and is in relationship with (Sauer et al. 2007). The need for a different framework considering the complexly networked human system, taking into account the role of mind and consciousness as well, is being felt. Realising that health cannot be limited to parts, modern medicine is now striving for an integrated and systems biology approach (Chaussabel 2004; Dinicola et al. 2011; Naylor and Chen 2010).

8.3 Quantum Worldview and Medical Science

By the nineteenth century, physicists felt everything in the universe including natural phenomena could be understood by Newtonian mechanics and expressed in quantitative mathematical terms. Within a few decades, however, a major revolution took place in the form of quantum mechanics, which studied atoms and beyond. The submicroscopic realm of these particles, it was found, was not deterministic but a very different one, where the particles can exist simultaneously in multiple states and possess a number of other seemingly contradictory properties defying the carefully built-up logic of classical physics. While the classical worldview assumes reality to be made of localisable material objects, the quantum world dealt with probabilities of existence and energy states (Alistair 1988; Feyman et al. 1965).

Quantum theory did not stop at being a theory of atomic phenomena but had repercussions for the macroscopic world as well. Challenging the conventional view of the physical world as a solid and stable material body, quantum physics brought in radical changes in the fundamental ideas about the nature of physical reality (Alistair 1988; Heisenberg 1958a). The universe came to be understood as a dynamic web of interconnected energy patterns, in which matter is a slowed-down form. In this web, no entities including humans are isolated, i.e. there is logically no such thing as a 'part' in the universe. Although at a macro-level the organisation and behaviour of the atomic world are stable giving the world an appearance of a solid form, the energies within this seemingly solid realm are not only moving but are also interconnected (Heisenberg 1958a). This new understanding of the universe as a stable pattern within which energy moves has brought about a change in the worldview – a very different concept of reality from that which grew out of the classical reductionistic physics. Quantum worldview has abandoned the idea of fundamental building blocks, which was central to the classical view.

The other radical shift brought in by quantum mechanics is the introduction of mind into the basic conceptual structure of physical reality. The central role a conscious observer plays has also made the quantum physical worldview radically different from the conventional one, where the observer has no active role but only a passive one (Stapp 2007). Interestingly, the practical successes of the Quantum theory, such as the applications of MRI, lasers, electron microscope, transistors, etc., have had significant impact in diagnostic and therapeutic medicine. The changes that have taken place in the worldview, however, have not translated into a new paradigm in Western medicine, which has persisted with the old reductionistic worldview model of Newtonian physics.

8.4 The Quantum and Vedic Worldviews

Questions about the nature of matter and reality have been raised in all civilisations and have been addressed by Indian seers of yore as well (Brunton 1939; Capra 1999; Jones 1986; Knapp 1990). These are elaborated in depth in *vedanta*, considered the culmination of *vedic* philosophies (Saraswati 2004) just as quantum physics is seen as the cutting edge of modern science. Though both these disciplines discuss the nature of reality, their approaches are from divergent viewpoints. According to *vedanta*, nature exists as a continuum and common principles underlie both the microcosm (individual) and macrocosm (universe) resulting in a unifying law binding everything in the universe. It goes on to say that everything in this universe has evolved from a single entity and is an extension of that, and so everything (including living beings) is interconnected and in a dynamic relationship (Saraswati 2004). The basic oneness of the universe is not only the essence of the *vedic* worldview but also one of the most important revelation of quantum physics. Like the *vedic* seers, the quantum physicists were also dealing with a nonsensory experience of reality through their studies on atomic particles, which provided them the first glimpses of the fundamental nature of matter. They found that underlying all physical matter is the intrinsically interconnected dynamic network of energy leaving nothing isolated in the universe (Heisenberg 1958a).

That there is an undeniable correlation between what physicists have discovered through observations, laboratory experiments and mathematical reasoning and what the Indian seers inferred from their observations, experiential experiments and logical reasoning has been commented by none other than Heisenberg, the architect of quantum mechanics. He says, 'After the conversations with Tagore about Indian philosophy, some of the ideas (of Quantum Physics) that had seemed so crazy suddenly made much more sense. That was a great help for me' (Capra 1989). He also says, 'All the same, some statements of ancient philosophy are rather near to those of modern science. This simply shows how far one can get by combining the ordinary experience of nature that we have without doing experiments with the untiring effort to get some logical order into this experience to understand it from general principles'.

Erwin Schrodinger, one of the fathers of quantum mechanics, also known for his deep interest in *Upanishad* (Capra 1989) had commented, 'the unity and continuity of *vedanta* are reflected in the unity and continuity of wave mechanics' (Gewali 2009; Schroedinger 1944). The logical point of contact between quantum theory and *vedic* thoughts, hence, lies in their worldviews and understanding of the nature of reality. Worldview has a bearing on the way a biological system is understood. We have seen the influence of classical worldview in Western medicine. The following sections outline the role of the integrative worldview of *veda* in Āyurveda.

8.5 Āyurveda

Long been the major healthcare system in India, the beginning of Āyurveda is lost in the mists of antiquity but is closely interwoven with the history and culture of the Indian sub-continent. Āyurvedic thoughts and methods have had a deep impact on the lifestyle of Indians. Its principles of healthy living, incorporated into day-to-day practices, are reflected in the daily activities, traditional cuisine using spices and medicinal ingredients, and even religious rituals of the Indians. In almost every household, there was (and still is) knowledge of āyurvedic treatment for common ailments. Āyurveda continues to have a pervasive influence in the daily life of Indians and has perhaps the longest unbroken health tradition in the world (Mukerjee 2006a; Varier 2005; Vidyanath and Nishteswar 2006).

Āyurveda is an applied science like Western medicine. While the basic sciences of the latter are physics and chemistry, the fundamental basis of Āyurveda are found in *darśana*, which are ancient Indian treatises on the physical and metaphysical aspects of the universe (Cowell and Gough 1978; Tigunait 1983). It is interesting to note the similarities between the words 'theory' and '*darśana*'. 'Theory' is derived from the Greek root word 'theoria' (*θεωρία*) meaning to 'view or observe'. Modern science has many theories, such as those of motion, gravity and evolution. A number of them are named after the scientists who first described them – e.g. Newton's laws of motion, Einstein's theory of relativity, etc. Although the word '*darśana*' has deeper philosophical meaning and implications, it also literally means 'to see or view'. As in modern science, the various '*darśana*' are also associated with names of those who formulated them: Kaṇāda's *Vaiśeṣika*, Gautamā's *Nyāya*, Jaimini's *Purva Mimāmsa*, Kapilā's *Sānkhya*, Patanjali's *Yogā* and Vyāsā's *Vedānta* (Cowell and Gough 1978; Muller 2003; Sandal 1999; Tigunait 1983).

The Indian seers of yore did not remain mere observers of nature but had theorised their observations using logical reasoning. *Sānkhya, Nyāya* and *Vaiśeṣika* explain the physical universe from a logical perspective, whereas *Vedanta* understands it from a spiritual perspective. *Nyāya* and *Vaiśeṣika* are best known for their rigorous analytical approaches and logical arguments (Tigunait 1983; Vidyabhushana 2003). *Vaiśeṣika* deals with the physical aspects of universe and their practical implications and interestingly postulates atomic nature of matter (Muller 2003). The concepts, logical reasoning and analytical methodologies of these materialistic schools have been used by Āyurveda to understand human body, health and ill health (Sharma and Dash 2001). While *yoga* focuses on the inner realms of humans, *Sānkhya* and *Vedānta* deal with creation, worldview, relationships and their philosophical implications (Saraswati 2004; Muller 2003; Nair 2005). These concepts have been used by Āyurveda to understand the various relationships governing life, its processes and also the relationship between humans and the cosmos (Rao 2002). Āyurveda has thus provided a practical platform, elevating these concepts from philosophical realms to that of science (Jayasundar 2008). The coherent theoretical framework drawn from these different *darśana* has given the base for Āyurveda's comprehensive knowledge of life. Āyurveda is essentially a science of life encompassing both health and ill health.

8.5.1 Impact of Vedic/Quantum Worldview on Āyurveda: Holism and Interconnectedness

Āyurveda is based on a concept of wholeness and unity that goes beyond a purely mechanistic view. Over the centuries, Āyurveda has collected enormous amounts of empirical data on which it has based all its theoretical generalisations. Though a number of theories are used to describe the human system, its viewpoint is predominantly functional (Jayasundar 2010). According to Āyurveda, the whole organism constitutes a functional entity. Function is a collective effort of several contributing factors ranging from structures, biochemical processes to various activities such as electrical, mental and even spiritual. Functional perspective is therefore inclusive, taking into consideration all the contributing factors including those of structures and biochemistry. Of the various theories, that of *tridoṣa* (*vāta, pitta* and *kapha*) runs as an undercurrent to the entire āyurvedic understanding of health and ill health, defining its functional perspective. How the quantum concept of interrelatedness is inbuilt into Āyurveda is best understood through the theory of *tridoṣa* and hence discussed in detail in this chapter.

The Sanskrit words *vāta, pitta* and *kapha* are referred to as '*doṣa*', meaning 'that which can become impaired and also has the potential to impair other tissues'. The *tridoṣa*, as they are collectively known, are concepts derived from nature (macrocosm) to explain human beings (microcosm). The functional/governing factors of *tridoṣa* were derived from those of the universe. *Suśruta* says,

> 'just like moon, sun and wind sustain the universe by their cold, heat and dispersion/movement, respectively, likewise *kapha*, *pitta* and *vāta* support the body with similar functions' (Suśruta Saṃhitā 21, 8 in Sharma 2004)

These principles extend to all living beings from the smallest to the largest. *Ćaraka* says (Sharma and Dash 2001)

> 'this is a science for well-being of all creatures' (Ćaraka Saṃhitā Sūtra Sthāna 1, 27 in Sharma and Dash 2001)
>
> 'these works were established on this earth for the good of all creatures' (Ćaraka Saṃhitā Sūtra Sthāna 1, 40 in Sharma and Dash 2001)

All biological systems from humans to animals and plants are thus described within this single framework of *tridoṣa*. For example, *vrkṣa* Āyurveda (āyurvedic botany) (Sadhale 1996; Sircar and Sarkar 1996) and *mṛga* Āyurveda (āyurvedic veterinary science) (Anjaria 1894; Mukerjee 2006b; Somvanshi 2006) use the same *tridoṣic* theory to explain their respective systems. It is, thus, a unifying theory encompassing all living organisms.

Interconnectedness Within the System

Āyurveda has grouped the vast information in the human system into three most fundamental functions and their contributing components/properties. These are *vāta*, *pitta* and *kapha*, indicating respectively, movement, transformation and support as well as growth (Jayasundar 2010). Figure 8.1 shows the classification and Figs. 8.2–8.4, the further sub-classifications of *doṣa* (Sharma and Dash 2001; Srikantamurthy 2005). It is to be noted that an exhaustive list of functions and parameters is not given in these figures. *Vāta*, *pitta* and *kapha* cover not only physiological but also psychological parameters such as enthusiasm, memory, wisdom

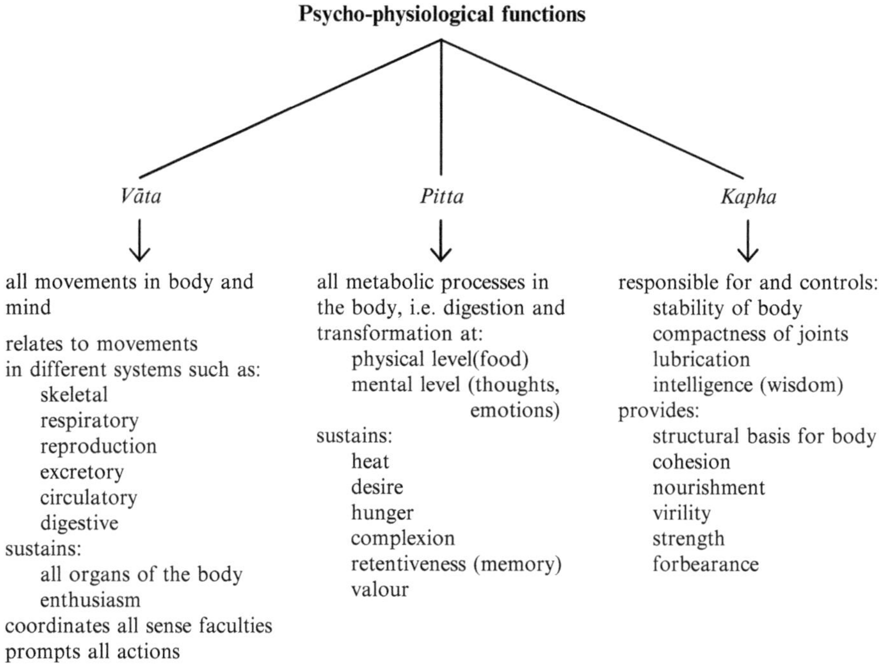

Fig. 8.1 Functional classification in Āyurveda (Source: Author, based on Ćaraka Saṃhitā and Ashtanga Samgraha)

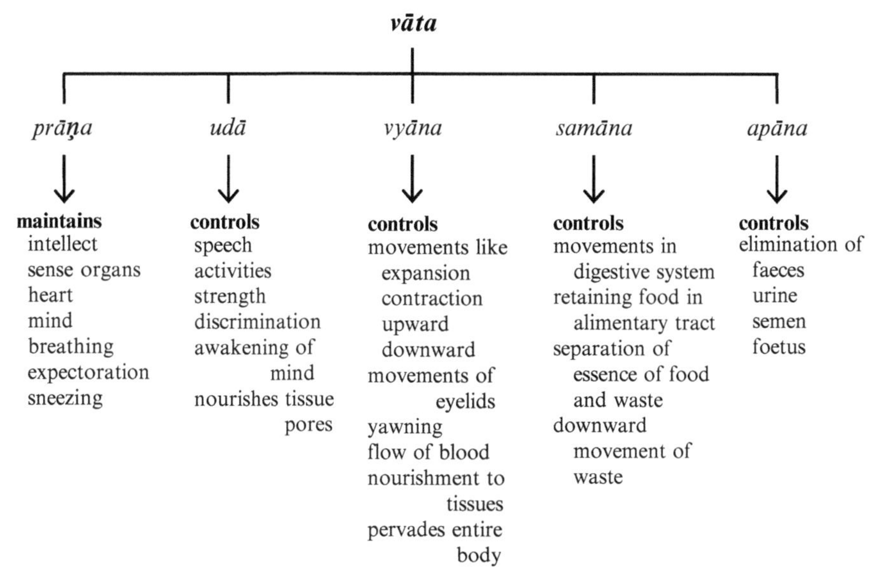

Fig. 8.2 Sub-classification of *vāta* (Source: Author, based on Ćaraka Saṃhitā and Ashtanga Samgraha)

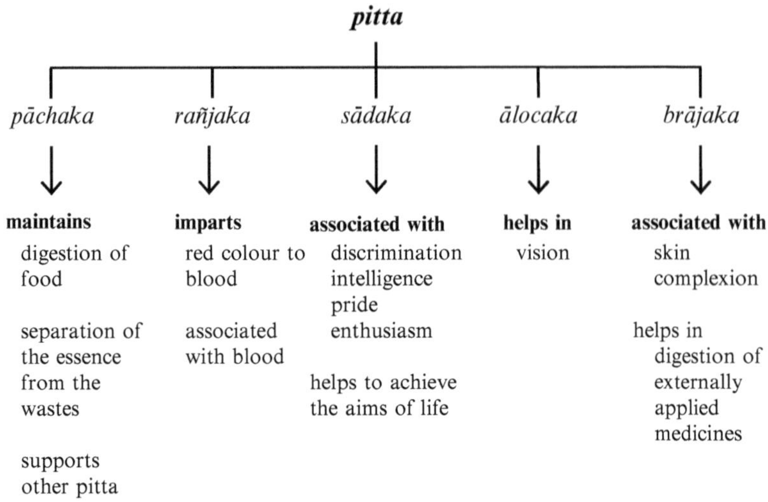

Fig. 8.3 Sub-classification of *pitta* (Source: Author, based on Ćaraka Saṃhitā and Ashtanga Samgraha)

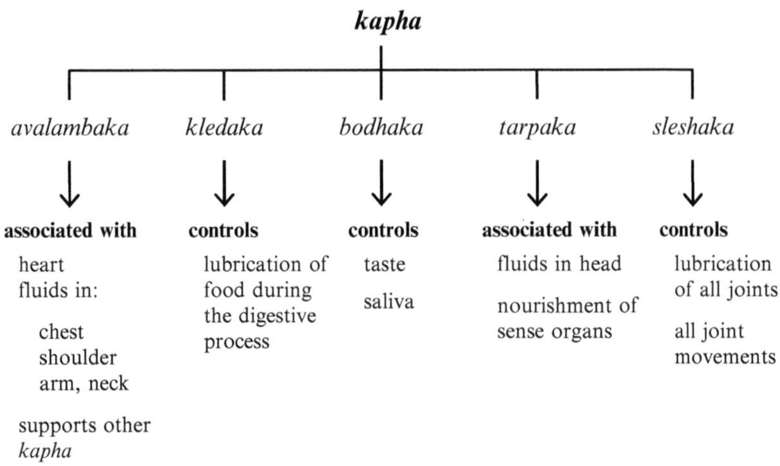

Fig. 8.4 Sub-classification of *kapha* (Source: Author, based on Ćaraka Saṃhitā and Ashtanga Samgraha)

and forbearance. *Vāta* indicates movement in the physical plane and also the flow/movement of thoughts in the mental space. Similarly *pitta* refers to digestion and transformation both at the physical and mental planes. The *tridoṣa*, thus, encompass both the physical and mental frame of the individual. Between them, the three *doṣa* and their 15 sub-classifications cover all psychophysiological functions in the body and the associated properties (refer to Figs. 8.5 and 8.6 for a list of these properties). Āyurveda also mentions the theory of three *guṇa*: *sattva, rajas and tamas*, which make up one's personality (Śārīra Sthāna, Sharma and Dash 2001).

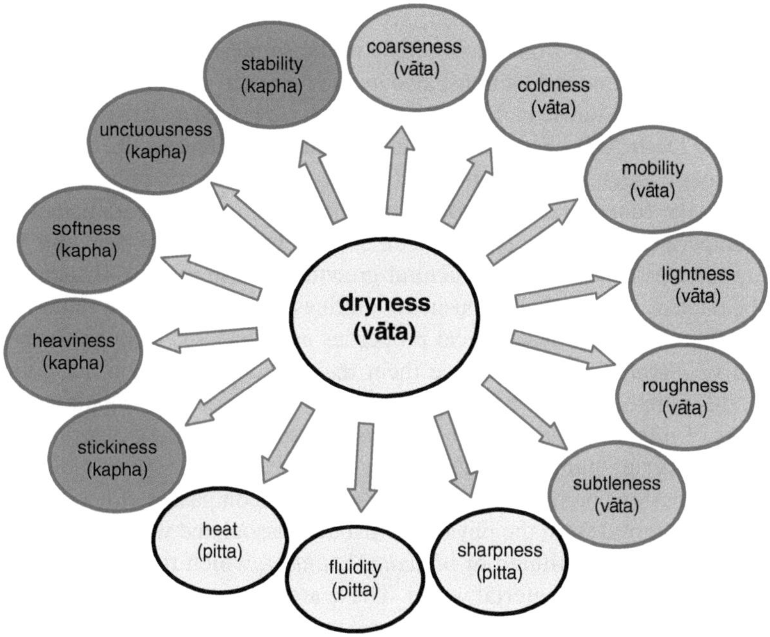

Fig. 8.5 Relation between the *vāta* factor of dryness and *pitta*, *kapha* and *vāta* parameters

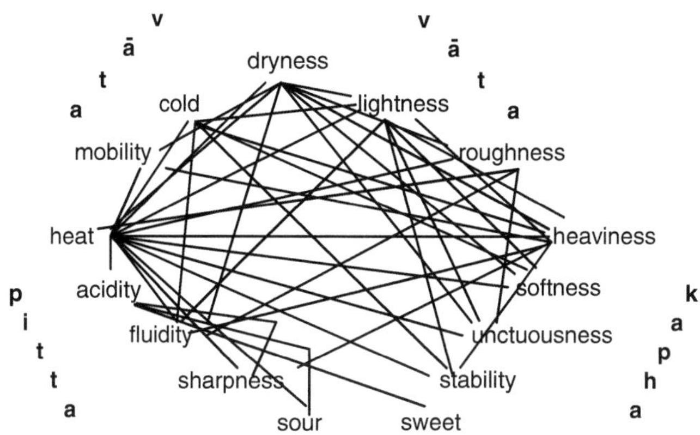

Fig. 8.6 Topological connectivities of *doṣa* factors

This is not discussed here since it is beyond the scope of this article. However, there is close association between the three *doṣa* and *guṇa* (Sūtra Sthāna, Sharma and Dash 2001).

Functions, unlike matter, cannot be reduced to fundamental entities like atoms and molecules. There is, hence, no functional hierarchy or basic building blocks in this āyurvedic perspective. The *doṣa*, i.e. the functions and the associated properties, exist at all levels – from macroscopic to the subtlest like cells. As mentioned, the *tridoṣa*, in addition to functions, also include physico-chemical and physiological parameters as shown in Figs. 8.5 and 8.6 (Jayasundar 2010; Sūtra Sthāna, Sharma and Dash 2001). For example, *vāta* includes parameters like dryness, lightness, coldness, roughness and subtleness, all of which influence movement. *Pitta*, in addition to the function of metabolic transformation, includes parameters such as heat (temperature), acidity (pH), unctuousness, penetrating power and fluidity. *Kapha* indicates cohesion and structural growth and also properties such as coldness, heaviness, softness, unctuousness, sliminess, stability and sweetness. These physico-chemical and physiological properties are expressed through the physical medium of *dhātu* (tissues) and give them their functionality. Without going into details, it is pointed out that while some of the properties are overlapping (e.g. unctuousness of *pitta* and *kapha*), some parameters such as dryness (*vāta*) and unctuousness (*kapha*) are mutually contradictory.

Just as functions include structures, *doṣa* also encompasses structural entities. This can be inferred from the physical attributes associated with *doṣa*. Moreover, the three *doṣa* are constituted of *pañcamahābhutā*, which refer to the five basic elements of the visible material world. These are earth, water, air, space and fire/light. While the first three refer to the three states of matter, namely, solid, liquid and gas, the latter two, i.e. space and fire/light, refer to other important elements and aspects of the visible world. While *vāta* is constituted of space and air, *pitta* is a combination of water and properties of fire and *kapha* is formed of earth and water. That the *doṣa* are physical entities is also inferred from their clinical usage. For example, during palliative treatment, *doṣa* are handled in the form of properties that have to be altered to maintain the *doṣic* balance. During elimination therapy, however, they are handled as physical substances (Chikitsa Sthāna, Sharma and Dash 2001). Thus, the *doṣic* functional model encompasses the structural aspects as well. *Doṣa* at one level are functional properties yet at another level are considered physical entities. They are dualistic on a pragmatic, therapeutic level but are non-dualistic on a conceptual level.

Within the System: The Non-linear Functional Network

Life, in Āyurveda, is viewed as a complex network of interrelated functions and properties and not as a system of chemicals or structures. Figure 8.5 is an illustrative example of how the *doṣa* are intra- and inter-connected. For example, the *vāta* factor dryness, is intra-connected with its own parameters and inter-connected with those of *pitta* and *kapha*. A change in dryness, therefore, is likely to effect changes in many other parameters. Āyurveda expresses these connections as a network of interdependent relationships, where the functioning of one influences many others.

Figure 8.6 showing the relational interdependence between some of these parameters also indicates the intricate interplay between them. It can be seen that some of the factors are connected to more than one parameter in this network. Consider a change in the factor 'dryness' associated with *vāta*. Dryness could occur at any level, from cell to organs to the entire system. At whichever level it occurs, the parameter can simultaneously reduce one *doṣa* and increase the other. For example, when dryness increases, there will be reduction in the 'unctuous' property of *kapha*, increase in the 'heat/temperature' of *pitta* and changes in a number of other parameters including those of roughness and lightness from its own category, i.e. *vāta*.

Interestingly, the resulting increase in temperature due to dryness will also cause changes in other parameters. In fact, each of these parametrical changes will affect the system in different ways leading ultimately to functional changes in movement, both at the initial level 'dryness' had occurred and also at other interacting levels. It is pertinent to note that Western medicine considers diseases such as keratoconjunctivitis sicca, xerostomia, atrophic vaginitis and xeroderma as 'medical dryness' (Berk 2008; Haslett et al. 2001; Petrone et al. 2002). The parameters interact at all levels and are continuously perturbed as a result of influences from other factors. These properties are entangled, i.e. they are dynamically interlinked to one another and form non-linear causal connections. The balance of the network depends on the dynamical behaviour of the parameters.

In a complex biological system, there are various levels of functions such as cellular, tissue, organ, etc., and multiple layers of integrative interaction to give functionality to the system. A change at a lower level can produce changes at other integrative levels and vice versa. For example, a mutation in a gene can be seen as a DNA change at a macromolecular level, a histological change at the tissue level and behavioural change at the organism level (Lobo 2008). Similarly, a change in one of the *doṣa* parameter at one level will be reflected at various levels and exercise a downward/upward control over the course of physiological events affecting the entire system since these are system properties applicable at all integrative levels. Through this *tridoṣa* theory, Āyurveda networks the complex human system as a dynamic web of relationships defining functions.

The framework of *tridoṣa* thus connects the entire system encompassing its inherent complexity with its various levels of interactions. The *doṣa* parameters are not a set of rigid linear causal connections but rather interdependent non-linear functional links encompassing also the physical entities. *Doṣa* thus offers a different perspective of human body and provides a conceptual framework very different from that of Western medicine. Āyurveda's view of life as a dynamic interrelationship between *vāta*, *pitta* and *kapha* gives it its distinctness in dealing with human system in an integrated and holistic way.

The key to health is for these parameters to maintain stability in the network despite perturbations, not only within the system, but also without. *Vagbhata* says,

> 'equilibrium of *doṣa* is health and their imbalance denotes disease' (Ashtanga Hridayam 1, 20 in Srikantamurthy 1999)

Health is indicated by the balanced interplay between the various functions and parameters, while disease is viewed as a system perturbation and a functional failure, because of which Āyurveda looks beyond the behaviour of individual parts and addresses the system properties in an effort to rebalance the system.

Āyurvedic treatment aims at restoration of the functional balance. The increase or decrease of *doṣa* is accompanied by symptoms, which are described in detail in āyurvedic texts. One can therefore infer the state of *doṣa* from the symptoms and take corrective measures to bring it back to equilibrium state. What is interesting is how Āyurveda has incorporated this concept of interrelatedness in a meaningful way into its diagnostic decision and therapeutic management. Integration of the theory of *tridoṣa* with clinical practice is discussed in detail by Jayasundar (2012a). Since the *doṣa* are non-linearly networked, Āyurveda's determinants of health and disease do not follow the linear causal pathways of Western medicine. Response of a non-linear system to variations in parameters is complex making causal thinking difficult (Albert 2007; Variano et al. 2004).

Within the System: The Structural Network

Despite the importance of functional classification, Āyurveda recognises the structural aspects of human body as well. It very clearly says all physical entities, including humans, are made of matter in five forms (*pañcamahābhūta*).

> 'according to this science, all matter is constituted of five *mahābhūta*; some are animate and some others inanimate' (Ćaraka Saṃhitā Sūtra Sthāna 26, 10 in Sharma and Dash 2001)

Substances endowed with consciousness are considered as much the products of matter as those without consciousness. This categorical statement and other similar assertions in *Ćaraka Saṃhitā* give clear indication that Āyurveda has a structural viewpoint as well. This is logical and understandable since the physical body, where the clinical symptoms ultimately manifest, is the only tangible reality to the treating physician. A physician cannot, therefore, but have a structural perspective as well.

Ćaraka says in no uncertain terms, 'Detailed knowledge of the human body is useful to the well-being of the individual. Understanding the components of the body provides knowledge regarding the factors responsible for its well-being. It is because of this that experts extol the knowledge of the details of the body' (Śārīra Sthāna, Sharma and Dash 2001). He goes onto say,

> 'when tissues (*dhātu*) in the body become discordant, then there is disease' (Ćaraka Saṃhitā Śārīra Sthāna 6, 3–4 in Sharma and Dash 2001)

It is important to note that surgical discipline, which gives importance to structures, was a highly developed branch in Āyurveda. *Suśruta*, the āyurvedic surgeon acknowledged as the father of surgery by Western medicine, emphasises the importance of anatomy and dissection and describes many surgical procedures (Chari 2003; Das 2001).

All the structural entities in the body are divided into minute units known as '*paramāṇu*', which like cells are numerous, subtle and beyond sensory perceptions (Ćaraka Saṃhitā Śārīra Sthāna 7, 17 in Sharma and Dash 2001). All the structural components (gross to subtle) are interconnected by *srotas*, a system of channels (Ćaraka Saṃhitā Vimāna Sthāna 5 in Sharma and Dash 2001). These are a complexly networked system for bio-transport of all essentials in the body such as fluids, nutrients, impulses and energies. The *srotas* system is a continuum connecting structures, both subtle and gross. Despite these, Āyurveda goes beyond a purely structural viewpoint. It considers life as a complex and coordinated interaction of various functions and properties, encompassing also subtle realms like mind and consciousness.

Within the System: Network of the Gross and Subtle

Āyurveda considers human being as a combination of two basic elements: consciousness (*cetana*) and inert matter (*jada*). The relationship between these two entities defines a human being. The realms within, hence, consist of not only physical and physiological but also mind and subtler levels of awareness/consciousness. Āyurveda says that the subtler levels within influence the physiology. By connecting these two realms, Āyurveda adopts a comprehensive view of life and health. While *Ćaraka* says,

> 'life is a combination of body, senses, mind and consciousness' (Ćaraka Saṃhitā Sūtra Sthāna 1, 42 in Sharma and Dash 2001),

Suśruta defines a healthy individual as,

> 'a healthy person is one whose *doṣa*, *dhātu* (structural entities) and metabolic end products are in equilibrium. And there must also be clarity in consciousness, senses and mind for a healthy state' (Suśruta Saṃhitā 15, 41 in Sharma 2004)

While the *tridoṣa* parameters (along with *triguṇa*) indicate the connection between the physical and mental planes, the theory of *pañcakośa*, used more extensively in yoga, deals in depth with the mental and subtler realms of existence. These are seen as comprising of discrete yet interdependent levels of awareness. Āyurveda and yoga are closely related disciplines. They share the common framework of *tridoṣa* theory, and Āyurveda supports concepts and applications of yoga. So, although the āyurvedic texts do not explicitly mention *pañcakośa*, it is understood that Āyurveda takes cognisance of this when it discusses mind, *buddhi* (intellect) and the role of different levels of consciousness in health and disease (Frawley 1998; Śārīra Sthāna, Sharma and Dash 2001). For example, Āyurveda considers mind (*manomayakośa*) and intellect (*vijnānamaya kośa*) to be separate (Ćaraka Saṃhitā Śārīra Sthāna 1, 23 in Sharma and Dash 2001). Interestingly, faulty understanding or mistake at the level of '*prañjā/buddhi*' (the capacity to understand and discriminate) is considered a major causative factor for diseases (discussed in the next section).

According to the theory of *pañcakośa*, there are five hierarchical levels of awareness/consciousness, from gross physical body (*annamaya kośa*) to the subtle spiritual body (*ānandamaya kośa*) (Aurobindo 1981; Johnsen 2003). Each level, from gross inwards, refers to a more refined dimension of awareness. The 5th level is the state where impurities of mind are removed and realisation of self is experienced.

What is of interest is the link between the subtlest level of consciousness (*ānandamaya kośa*) and the gross physical body (*annamaya kośa*) through the intervening layers of *prānamaya*, *manomaya* and *vijñānamaya kośa*. These levels are progressive in scale of subtility and refinement. Moving from the gross to the subtle helps one to develop discriminatory wisdom and detachment, enabling a shift towards a more happy and productive and less destructive realms of existence. The direction of evolution is towards subtler/higher levels of awareness culminating in unity with the infinite, resulting in happiness and freedom from causes of suffering.

The functions and purpose of each layer and their relation with other levels are stated in the following lines from *Yogavāsiṣta* (Murthy 2002):

> 'For one without discrimination (of what is right and wrong),
> application of sciences is a burden;
>
> For one with knowledge but unwilling to use it properly,
> the knowledge itself is a burden;
>
> For one who is agitated,
> mind is a burden;
>
> For one who does not understand oneself,
> body itself is a burden'.

A mere possession of mental faculties and knowledge will not lead to one's well-being unless accompanied with right values and thinking to sustain harmony within and without. Awareness of oneself is necessary for health.

Āyurveda refers to a healthy individual as '*svastha*', which is defined as '*sve tiṣtati iti svastha*': one who is established in oneself. Implicit in this is the fact that lack of awareness will lead to impaired knowledge, which Āyurveda points out is a causative factor for diseases (Ćaraka Saṃhitā Nidāna Sthāna 1, 3 in Sharma and Dash 2001). Any change in perception that takes place in *buddhi* is reflected in the body/physiology. This is why training the intellect is considered important in maintaining health. Regimens, which influence *buddhi*, are considered as important as diet and behavioural routines. It helps bring mind under control so one does not make errors in judgement and action. There are important *chants* like *Gayatri mantra* (*GM*), which help train the intellect and keep it in a healthy condition by their sound and content. That GM has a measurable effect on brain metabolites has been demonstrated using MR spectroscopy by Jayasundar and Rajshekar (2000). Āyurveda clearly considers mind and body to be intrinsically linked with consciousness, which acts as the fulcrum of health. *Ćaraka* says, 'mind is the link between consciousness and physical body' (Ćaraka Saṃhitā Śārīra Sthāna 2, 13 in Sharma and Dash 2001). Āyurveda thus links and networks the gross (physical body) and subtle (mind and consciousness).

Figure 8.7 shows in a nutshell how the physical, physiological, mental and subtler domains within the body are intra- and inter-connected. Each domain is not only networked within but also connected to others. For example, *srotas* networks the structures, *doṣa* the physiology, *guṇa* the mind and *pañcakośa* the levels of consciousness. The structures and physiology are connected via *doṣa and srotas*,

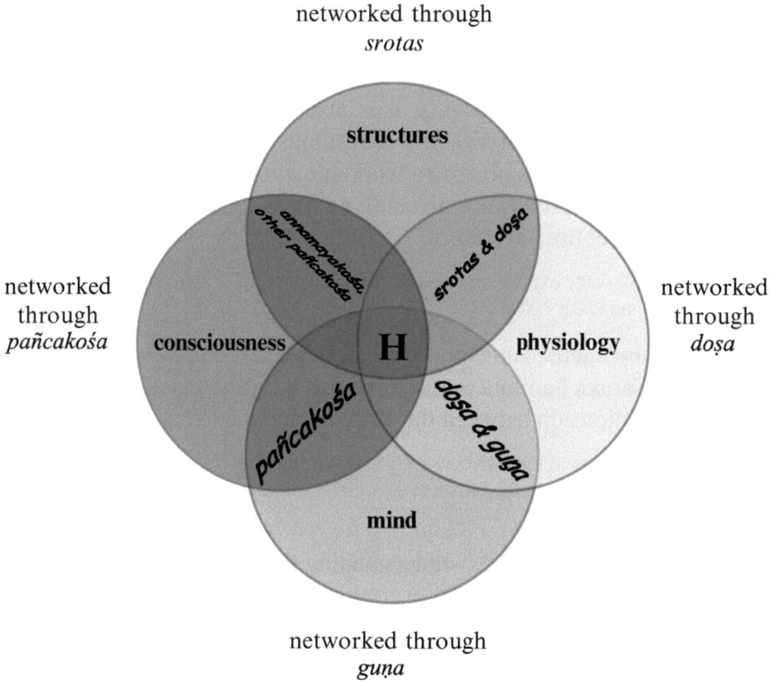

Fig. 8.7 Intra- and inter- connections in the network of structures, physiology, mind and consciousness. H refers to human being

physiology and mind through *doṣa* and *guṇa* and mind and consciousness through *pañcakośa*. The consciousness is linked to the physical body (structures) through its first level of awareness. So, each domain while acting as a network within itself is also networked with others. They form several interlocking networks making a coherent whole. The domains, which can be considered as subnetworks, are not functionally insulated, so failure or imbalance in one affects the entire human system. This highlights the centrality of the quantum concept of interconnectedness in Āyurveda.

Interconnectedness Outside the System

Individual and the Universe

Human being is not a separate entity dissociated from the universe but is like an open system. In other words, there is exchange/interaction with the environment and also the universe. The subtlest level of consciousness (*ānandamaya kośa*) in the human is linked to the cosmic consciousness, and yoga helps one connect these two (Saraswati 1998; Ćaraka Saṃhitā Śārīra Sthāna I, 155 and V, 21 in Sharma and

Dash 2001). In this connected state, the external universe is no longer considered external, the internal no longer internal and everything is seen as an undivided whole, i.e. there is no boundary. Thus, not only is the physiology linked to the microcosmic world of consciousness, it is also connected through the levels of awareness (*kośa*) to the macrocosmic consciousness. These theories (*tridoṣa, triguṇa and pañcakośa*) thus provide a workable interface between the microcosm (individual) and the macrocosm (universe). *Ćaraka* says the individual exists as a continuum with the entire universe-

> 'the whole universe is the expansion of one's consciousness' (Ćaraka Saṃhitā Śārīra Sthāna 5, 20 in Sharma and Dash 2001)

Ćaraka calls the microcosmic consciousness as '*viśvarūpa*', meaning prototype of the universe (Ćaraka Saṃhitā Śārīra Sthāna 4, 8 in Sharma and Dash 2001), and establishes the relationship between the individual and universe by saying,

> 'all the manifest objects in the universe are present in the individual and all that is present in the individual manifests in the universe as well' (Ćaraka Saṃhitā Śārīra Sthāna 4, 13 in Sharma and Dash 2001)

Implicit in these statements is the understanding that the objective world is potentially inherent in the individual, and everything within or outside is related to the subject from which they expand. The relevance of this knowledge in the context of medicine is also explained by *Ćaraka*. He says,

> 'this (the above-mentioned) is true knowledge and realisation of this leads to serenity of mind' (Ćaraka Saṃhitā Śārīra Sthāna V, 6, 20–21 in Sharma and Dash 2001)

Serenity of mind in turn will lead to harmony and health.

Individual and the Environment

Āyurveda recognises that the health of an individual is dependent and intertwined with that of the environment and advises a harmonious relationship between the two. Maintenance of such a harmony is essential to the health of a living organism, be it human, animal or plant. *Doṣa* increases or decreases naturally during different seasons (seasonal rhythms) and also during the course of the day (e.g. diurnal cycle) and influences one's health. This interconnectedness of individual with the environment finds practical expression in various āyurvedic concepts such as causative factors during epidemics (Ćaraka Saṃhitā Vimāna Sthāna 3, 4 in Sharma and Dash 2001) and daily and seasonal regimens (Sūtra Sthāna, Sharma and Dash 2001). These regimens, consisting of dos and don'ts for diet and activities, take care of the response of the body to outside changes and establish a functional harmony between the individual and environment. While personal interface with macrocosmic consciousness is through yoga, that with the physical environment is through these regimens, which ensure both individual and community health.

The case of a 45-year-old patient (personal communication 2009) is discussed here to illustrate this point – the patient was suffering from heavy bouts of cough and cold every spring season for nearly 6 years and was on heavy antibiotics during the affected period. From an āyurvedic perspective, this *kapha*-related seasonal problem was identified as indulgence in diet and activities incompatible with spring season, during which there is a general aggravated manifestation of *kapha* in everybody. The patient had been indulging in *kapha*-aggravating foods such as citrus fruits, yoghurt and fruit juice, all of which are incompatible with spring season. The patient's problem was addressed simply by correcting the diet and activities. Post intervention, the patient has faced four spring seasons without recurrence of the problem. This example shows how a person's well-being is connected to environmental changes, and how Āyurveda's preventive routines can be effectively used to avoid seasonal diseases. Āyurveda is peppered with information on how to achieve welfare for all by working in conjunction with nature. It is a way of life contributing to harmonious health within and without (Jayasundar 2012b).

8.6 Quantum Framework of Āyurveda

Is Āyurveda an ancient or a state-of-the-art science? It is an interesting question that can be addressed by looking backwards from today's vantage point of modern scientific knowledge. Quantum physics, considered the cutting edge of Western science has exposed concepts similar to those discussed in the Indian knowledge system of *veda* (Capra 1999; Jones 1986; Talbot 1993). Two quantum concepts that find practical expression in Āyurveda are interconnectedness and the role of consciousness. The first concept relates to the fundamental interrelatedness of all phenomena, and the dynamic and interdependent nature of reality.

The central core idea of Āyurveda is that everything within (microcosm) and without (macrocosm) the human body is interrelated and their balance denotes health or ill health. The whole existence is like a network, where a change in one part is likely to perturb the entire system. Āyurveda has integrated and implemented this concept through theories like *tridoṣa* and offers a practical method to sustain the relationship between individual and the universe. Interconnectedness is part of the terminology of both quantum and *vedic*/āyurvedic worldviews which sees oneness in all things. Āyurveda's paradigm thus is closer to the quantum physical worldview.

The other quantum concept is the role of consciousness. An observer is critical to the quantum concepts since behaviour of a quantum system cannot be predicted without the involvement of this macroscopic conscious entity. There is, thus, an interaction between observer and the observed in the microcosmic world of atoms, where an object does not exist independent of its observer. Human consciousness entered the realm of physics through this involvement of a conscious observer. John Wheeler's famous statement was 'We are not only observers. We are participators' (Wheeler 1990). Although the reference was initially to a conscious observer, later on it was suggested by David Bohm that this consciousness was at a deeper level and intrinsic to matter (Bohm and Hiley 1993; Penrose 1987).

Human experience was thus elevated from the role of a detached observer in classical physics to that of a participatory observer in quantum physics. As Heisenberg notes in 'The Copenhagen Interpretation of Quantum Theory',

> 'our scientific work in physics consists in asking questions about nature in the language that we possess and trying to get an answer from experiment by the means at our disposal. In this way quantum theory reminds us, as Bohr has put it, of the old wisdom that when searching for harmony in life one must never forget that in the drama of existence we are ourselves both players and spectators. It is understandable that in our scientific relation to nature our own activity becomes very important when we have to deal with parts of nature into which we can penetrate only by using the most elaborate tools.' (Adams 2000)

Consciousness is an integral part of health in Āyurveda, which defines health as a complete balance of body, mind and soul/consciousness. By including mind and consciousness, Āyurveda has included the invisible realms within human body in its understanding of health and disease. Just like the quantum model makes consciousness causally effective (Heisenberg 1958b), Āyurveda also considers consciousness causally effective in the emergence of disease (Ćaraka Saṃhitā Sūtra Sthāna 8, 13 in Sharma and Dash 2001; Ćaraka Saṃhitā Śārīra Sthāna 1, 35, 39–42 in Sharma and Dash 2001). Consciousness and physical body are considered entangled in Āyurveda. Although quantum physics' usage of the term 'consciousnesses' may not be the same as that in Āyurveda, the parallels and the inclusion in both are interesting. The consciousness attributed to in quantum physics could refer to one of the '*pañcakośa*' levels of awareness – *manomaya* or *vijnānamaya kośa*.

Āyurveda in the way it was originally developed and practised understood the interaction between consciousness and physical body to be a major factor in creating health or illness. The main cause of disease in Āyurveda is '*Prajnāparāda*', the impairment of knowledge or fault of the intellect, a mistake at the level of the inner consciousness (one of the *kośa*) (Ćaraka Saṃhitā Nidāna Sthāna 1, 3 in Sharma and Dash 2001). It refers to the deliberate, wilful indulgence in unhealthy practices leading to imbalance in *doṣa* resulting in disease. Āyurveda's concept that one's thoughts create health or ill health in the physical body resonates with that of quantum physics which says that our thoughts create the physical reality (Alistair 1988; Stapp 2007). One's perception of the world and the consequent behaviour affects the physiology to an extent that errors in perception can lead to psychosomatic disorders. Āyurveda emphasises the individual's ability to shape his/her health based on how they choose to think and behave. The physical event in gross body and psychic event in the mental space are seen in Āyurveda as two correlated events.

There are also other interesting conceptual parallels between Āyurveda and quantum concepts. For example, quantum physics highlights the fact that while there is certainly a matter-based classical universe, there is also a mind-based quantum universe. Nature is a continuum having both mechanical as well as quantum aspects and quantum theory underscores this dualistic aspect of nature. According to Āyurveda, human as an entity has two states, namely consciousness and inertness, with two distinguishable aspects – dispersed and localised. The dispersed aspect is mind and localised state is body. But both these states have a common origin and hence are related to each other and incessantly dynamic. Āyurveda says mind and matter exist in a continuum. It has incorporated this concept by considering the human body as mechanistic at one level and as levels of consciousness in the subtler realms. Mind and consciousness are thus inbuilt into āyurvedic's understanding of humans. *Ćaraka* says, 'mind, consciousness and body are like a tripod (for sentient beings) and constitutes the subject matter of Āyurveda' (Ćaraka Saṃhitā Sūtra Sthāna 1, 46–47 in Sharma and Dash 2001). The seemingly different worlds of gross (localised) and subtle (dispersed) are thus connected and networked in Āyurveda.

8.7 Concluding Thoughts

The fundamental difference that exists between Western medicine and Āyurveda largely stems from their worldviews – the former focuses on parts, while Āyurveda on the system. The worldviews, rather than being merely topics of interest in metaphysics, have influenced the perspectives of biology and medicine both in Western medical system and Āyurveda. Classical physics remains an excellent approximation at macroscopic level and Newtonian reductionism continues to be a very successful approach in Western medicine for in-depth understanding of the system components. However, by omitting all references to mental realities, classical physics has also produced a logical disconnect between the physical and mental realms. The necessity for a system perspective in clinical medicine has now been recognised. Science now acknowledges that human system cannot be explained in purely deterministic and objective terms. It confirms that psychological effects are not restricted to the psyche but get translated into the physical plane and plays a crucial role in health and disease (Dubovsky 2008; Kubzansky and Thurston 2007). Although the role of mind in health and disease is being increasingly acknowledged in conventional Western medicine, it is yet to be successfully incorporated into its health and therapeutic managements. Psychoneuroimmunology is still a new medical speciality in modern medicine (Ader 2007).

Quantum physics has indicated a shift from the classical, reductionistic worldview where consciousness has no role, to a holistic and non-deterministic concept of nature with a definite role for consciousness. The detached, objective observer of classical physics is actually consciously involved in the world he/she observes. The concept of consciousness, however, finds no place in the current working of biomedicine, which connects physiology to structures in contrast to the 'physiology to consciousness' connection in Āyurveda. In the Western approach, everything translates into chemical reactions at body level and therefore has to be treated from a chemistry point of view. Biology is understood in terms of biochemistry and cellular mechanics.

It is important to note that the basic logic system in Āyurveda has also been derived by observing nature at the macroscopic level as in classical physics. Āyurveda, while accepting the reality of gross physical body, also emphasises the interplay of forces beneath the physical structures and has evolved a practical method of handling these through the functional theory of *tridoṣa*. However, since Āyurveda is based on doctrines that understand the universe from both physical and spiritual perspectives, it also encompasses mind and consciousness in its concept of health and disease management. In fact, it uses both physical and metaphysical methods such as yoga and *mantra* in its therapeutic management. Āyurveda understands the human system as a network of relationships that includes consciousness in a fundamental way.

Interconnectedness being an integral part of its understanding of health and disease, Āyurveda goes beyond linear relationships and single causative factors for disease. It uses multiple parameters from different realms within and without the system to achieve a holistic perspective of the individual and brings into focus the contextual milieu responsible for a disease. By incorporating the *vedic* worldview, which is similar to that of quantum physics, Āyurveda has integrated the concept of interdependent interconnectedness in humans, thus opening the door to an interesting dialogue between quantum physics and āyurvedic approach to health and disease. While Western medicine's paradigm lies outside the quantum concepts of interconnectedness and the role of consciousness, Āyurveda's unifying approach lies within this quantum framework. It is a health model that connects gross and subtle within the body, individual and environment, and human and cosmos.

References

Adams, S. (2000). *Frontiers: Twentieth century physics*. London: Taylor and Francis.

Ader, R. (2007). *Psychoneuroimmunology*. New York: Elsevier, Inc.

Albert, R. (2007). Network inference, analysis, and modelling in systems biology. *The Plant Cell, 19*, 3327–3338.

Alistair, R. (1988). *Quantum physics: Illusion or reality*. London: Cambridge University Press.

Anjaria, J. (1894). *Hasti Āyurveda. Treatise on elephant medicine*. Kanhangad: Anand Ashram.

Aurobindo. (1981). *The Upanishads – Texts, translation and commentaries*. Pondicherry: Sri Aurobindo Ashram.

Avenell, A., Broom, J., Brown, T. J., Poobalan, A., Aucott, L., Stearns, S. C., Smith, W. C. S., Jung, R. T., Campbell, M. K., & Grant, A. M. (2004). Systematic review of the long term effects and economic consequences of treatments for obesity and implications for health improvement. *Health Technology Assessment, 8*, 1–182.

Beresford, M. J. (2010). Medical reductionism: Lessons from the great philosophers. *Quarterly Journal of Medicine, 103*, 721–724.

Berk, L. (2008). Systemic pilocarpine for treatment of xerostomia. *Expert Opinion on Drug Metabolism & Toxicology, 4*, 1333–1340.

Bickle, J. (2003). *Philosophy and neuroscience: A ruthlessly reductive account*. Dordrecht: Kluwer.

Bishop, F. L., & Lewith, G. T. (2010). Who uses CAM? A narrative review of demographic characteristics and health factors associated with CAM use. *Evidence-Based Complementary and Alternative Medicine, 7*, 11–28.

Bohm, D., & Hiley, B. J. (1993). *The undivided universe: An ontological interpretation of quantum theory*. London: Routledge.

Brunton, P. (1939). *Indian philosophy and modern culture*. London: Rider & Co.

Burtt, E. A. (1952). *The metaphysical foundations of modern science*. New York: Humanities Press.

Butterfield, H. (1997). *The origins of modern science*. New York: Free Press.

Capra, F. (1989). *Uncommon wisdom: Conversations with remarkable people*. New York: Simon and Schuster.

Capra, F. (1999). *The Tao of physics: An exploration of the parallels between modern physics and eastern mysticism* (4th ed.). New York: Shambhala Publication.

Chari, P. S. (2003). Suśruta and our heritage. *Indian Journal of Plastic Surgery, 36*, 4–13.

Chaussabel, D. (2004). Biomedical literature mining: Challenges and solutions in the Omics' era. *American Journal of Pharmacogenomics, 4*, 383–393.

Conrad, L. I., Neve, M., Nutton, V., Porter, R., & Wear, A. (1995). *The western medical tradition: 800 BC to 1800 AD*. Cambridge: Cambridge University Press.

Cottingham, J., Stoothoff, R., Kenny, A., & Murdoch, D. (1988). *The philosophical writings of Descartes in 3 vols*. Cambridge: Cambridge University Press.

Cowell, E. B., & Gough, A. E. (1978). *Review of the different systems of Hindu philosophy*. Varanasi: Chowkhamba Sanskrit Series Office.

Das, S. (2001). Suśruta, the pioneer urologist of antiquity. *The Journal of Urology, 165*, 1405–1408.

Davidovits, P. (2007). *Physics in biology and medicine* (3rd ed.). New York: Academic.

Dean, C. (2005). *Death by modern medicine*. New York: Ashtree Publication.

Dinicola, S., D'Anselmi, F., Pasqualato, A., Proietti, S., Lisi, E., Cucina, A., & Bizzarri, M. (2011). A systems biology approach to cancer: Fractals, attractors, and nonlinear dynamics. *OMICS, A Journal of Integrative Biology, 15*, 1–12.

Dubovsky, S. (2008). Emotional health = heart health. *Journal Watch Psychiatry, 128*, 1–2.

Feyman, R. P., Leighton, R., & Sands, M. (1965). *The Feyman lectures on physics*. Reading: Addison-Wesley.

Frawley, D. (1998). *Yoga and Āyurveda*. Kandern: Narayana verlag GmbH.

Gandhi, T. K., Weingart, S. N., Borus, J., Seger, A. C., Peterson, J., Burdick, E., Seger, D. L., Shu, K., Federico, F., Leape, L. L., & Bates, D. W. (2003). Adverse drug events in ambulatory care. *The New England Journal of Medicine, 348*, 1556–1564.

Gewali, S. (2009). *What is India? Know the answer from the world reknowned intellectual giants*. Shillong: Academic Publications.

Goossens, H., Ferech, M., Stichele, R. V., & Elseviers, M. (2005). Outpatient antibiotic use in Europe and association with resistance: A cross-national database study. *Lancet, 9459*, 579–587.

Haldane, R., & Ross, G. R. T. (1911). *The Philosophical works of Descartes. Vol. I: Discourse on method* (Part VI, pp. 119–120). Cambridge: Cambridge University Press.

Haslett, C., Chilvers, E. R., Hunter, J. A. A., & Boon, N. A. (2001). *Davidson's principles and practice of medicine*. London: Churchill Livingston.

Hawkey, P. M., & Jones, A. M. (2009). The changing epidemiology of resistance. *The Journal of Antimicrobial Chemotherapy, 64*(Suppl. 1), i3–i10.

Heisenberg, W. (1958a). The representation of nature in contemporary physics. *Daedalus, 87*, 95–108.

Heisenberg, W. (1958b). *Physics and philosophy*. New York: Harper.

Illich, I. (2003). Medical nemesis. *Journal of Epidemiology and Community Health, 57*, 919–922.

Ito, M. (2006). Cerebellar circuitry as a neuronal machine. *Progress in Neurobiology, 78*, 272–303.

Jayasundar, R. (2008). Quantum physics, Āyurveda and spirituality. In S. C. Mishra & S. Ghosh (Eds.), *Science and spiritual quest* (pp. 11–28). Kolkata: Bhaktivedanta Institute.

Jayasundar, R. (2009). Health and disease: Distinctive approaches to biomedicine and Āyurveda. *Leadership Medica, 15*, 6–21.

Jayasundar, R. (2010). Āyurveda: A distinctive approach to health and disease. *Current Science, 98*, 908–914.

Jayasundar, R. (2012a). Contrasting approaches to health and disease: Āyurveda and biomedicine. In V. Sujata & L. Abraham (Eds.), *Medicine, state and society: Indigenous medicine and medical pluralism in contemporary India* (pp. 37–58). Delhi: Orient BlackSwan.

Jayasundar, R. (2012b). Healthcare, the ayurvedic way. *Indian Journal of Medical Ethics, 9*, 177–179.
Jayasundar, R., & Rajshekar, K. (2000). A preliminary study of the shift in Left/Right biochemical asymmetry by conscious mental routine. In J. R. Isaac & K. Batra (Eds.), *Cognitive systems: Reviews & previews* (pp. 667–674). Delhi: Phoenix Publishing House.
Johnsen, L. (2003). Layers of being: Uncovering your inner self. *Yoga International, 2*, 78–85.
Jones, R. H. (1986). *Science and mysticism: A comparative study of western natural science, Theravada Buddhism and Advaita*. London/Toronto: Bucknell University Press.
Joyner, M. J. (2011). Giant sucking sound: Can physiology fill the intellectual void left by the reductionists? *Journal of Applied Physiology, 111*, 335–342.
Kane, S. A. (2009). *Introduction to physics in modern medicine* (2nd ed.). New York: CRC Press, Taylor & Francis Group.
Keller, E. (2000). *The century of the gene*. Cambridge, MA: Harvard University Press.
Kemper, K. J., Vohra, S., & Walls, R. (2008). The use of complementary and alternative medicine in pediatrics. *Pediatrics, 122*, 1374–1386.
Knapp, S. (1990). *The secret teachings of the Vedas*. Detroit: The World Relief Network.
Kubzansky, L. D., & Thurston, R. C. (2007). Emotional vitality and incident coronary heart disease: Benefits of healthy psychological functioning. *Archives in Psychiatry, 64*, 1393–1401.
Lazarou, J., Pomeranz, B., & Corey, P. (1998). Incidence of adverse drug reactions in hospitalized patients. *Journal of the American Medical Association, 279*, 1200–1205.
Libet, B. (2003). Can conscious experience affect brain activity? *Journal of Consciousness Studies, 10*, 24–28.
Lobo, I. (2008). Biological complexity and integrative levels of organisation. *Nature Education, 1*, 1–3.
Mackenbach, J. P. (2006). The origins of human disease: A short story on where diseases come from. *Journal of Epidemiology and Community Health, 60*, 81–86.
Miller, K. (2011). *Biomechanics of the brain*. New York: Springer.
Moore, T. J., Psaty, B. M., & Furberg, C. D. (1998). Time to act on drug safety. *Journal of the American Medical Association, 279*, 1571–1573.
Morandi, A., Tosto, C., Sartori, G., Roberti di Sarsina, P. (2011). Advent of a Link between Ayurveda and modern health science: The Proceedings of the First International Congress on Ayurveda, "Ayurveda: The Meaning of Life-Awareness, Environment, and Health", Milan, Italy, March 21–22, 2009. *Evidence Based Complementary and Alternative Medicine, 2011*, 929083. doi: 10.1155/2011/929083. Epub 2010 Oct 17.
Morange, M. (2001). A successful form of reductionism. *The Biochemist, 23*, 37–39.
Mukerjee, G. N. (2006a). *History of Indian medicine* (3 vols.). Delhi: Chaukhamba Sanskrit Pratisthan.
Mukerjee, G. N. (2006b). *History of Indian medicine* (Vol. 2, pp. 202–252). Delhi: Chaukhamba Sanskrit Pratisthan.
Muller, F. M. (2003). *Six systems of Indian philosophy; Samkhya and Yoga; Nyaya and Vaiseshika*. Montana: Kessinger Publishing LLC.
Murthy, P. N. (2002). *Commentary on yoga vāsishta*. Delhi: Bhavans Books.
Nair, P. K. S. (2005). *The Sankhya system*. Delhi: New Bharatiya Book Corporation.
Naylor, S., & Chen, N. Y. (2010). Unravelling human complexity and disease with systems biology and personalised medicine. *Personalised Medicine, 7*, 275–289.
Nutton, V. (2004). *Ancient medicine*. London: Routledge.
Penrose, R. (1987). Quantum physics and conscious thought. In B. J. Hiley & F. D. Peat (Eds.), *Quantum implications: Essays in honour of David Bohm*. London/New York: Routledge and Kegan Paul.
Petrone, D., Condemi, J. J., Fife, R., Gluck, O., Cohen, S., & Dalgin, P. (2002). A double-blind, randomized, placebo-controlled study of cevimeline in Sjögren's syndrome patients with xerostomia and keratoconjunctivitis sicca. *Arthritis Rheumatology, 46*, 748–754.
Rao, R. M. (2002). *Padartha Vijnanam*. Vijayawada: Suśruta Publishers.
Sadhale, N. (Translator). (1996). *Surapala's Vriksha Āyurveda: The science of plant life by Surapala*. Secunderabad: Asian Agri-History Foundation.

Sandal, M. L. (1999). *Mimamsa Sutras of Jaimini*. Delhi: Motilal Banarasidas.
Saraswati, N. (1998). Pañca Kośa: The five sheaths of the human personality. *Spectrum: The Journal of the British Wheel of Yoga, 4*, 7–9.
Saraswati, D. (2004). *Exploring Vedanta*. Coimbatore: Arsha Vidya centre, Research and Publication.
Sauer, U., Heinemann, M., & Zamboni, N. (2007). Getting close to the whole picture. *Science, 316*, 550–551.
Schroedinger, E. (1944). *What is life? The physical aspect of the living cell with mind and matter and autobiographical sketches*. Cambridge: Cambridge University Press.
Shahri, N. M., & Hagemann, N. (2011). Understanding drug resistance to biologic therapy. Resistance – the true face of biological defiance. *Rheumatology, 11*, 1–10.
Sharma, P. V. (Translator). (2004). *Suśruta Saṃhitā* (Sutra Sthana, Vol. 1). Varanasi: Chaukhamba Visvabharati.
Sharma, R. K., & Dash, B. (Translators). (2001). *Ćaraka Saṃhitā*. Varanasi: Chaukhamba Sanskrit Series Office.
Sircar, N. N., & Sarkar, R. (1996). *Vrksha Āyurveda of Parashara*. Delhi: Indian Books Centre.
Somvanshi, R. (2006). Shalihotra – Haya Āyurveda in veterinary medicine and animal keeping in ancient India. *Asian Agri-History, 10*, 133–146.
Srikantamurthy, K. R. (Translator). (1999). *Ashtanga Hridayam of Vagbhata*. Varanasi: Krishnadas Academy.
Srikantamurthy, K. R. (Translator). (2005). *Ashtanga Samgraha of Vagbhata*. Varanasi: Chaukambha Orientalia.
Stapp, H. P. (2007). *Mindful universe: Quantum mechanics and the participating observer*. Berlin: Springer.
Talbot, M. (1993). *Mysticism and the new physics*. USA: Arkana.
Tigunait, P. R. (1983). *Seven systems of Indian philosophy*. Haridwar: The Himalayan International Institute of Yoga.
Van Regenmortel, M. H. V., & Hull, D. (2002). *Promises and limits of reductionism in the biomedical sciences*. Chichester: Wiley.
Variano, E. A., McCoy, J. H., & Lipson, H. (2004). Networks, dynamics and modularity. *Physics Review Letters, 92*(188701), 1–4.
Varier, N. V. K. (2005). *History of Āyurveda* (Kottakkal Āyurveda series: 56). Kottakkal: Arya Vaidya Sala.
Ventura, H. O. (2000). Giovanni Battista Morgagni and the foundation of modern medicine. *Clinical Cardiology, 23*, 792–794.
Vidyabhushana, S. C. (2003). *Nyaya Darshana of Gotama*. Delhi: New Bharatiya Book Corporation.
Vidyanath, R., & Nishteswar, K. (2006). *A handbook of history of Āyurveda*. Varanasi: Chowkambha Sanskrit Series Office.
Wade, C., Chao, M., Kronenberg, F., Cushman, L., & Kalmuss, D. (2008). Medical pluralism among American women: Results of a national survey. *Journal of Women's Health, 17*, 829–840.
Wheeler, J. A. (1990). Information, physics, quantum: The search for links. In W. H. Zurek (Ed.), *Complexity, entropy and the physics of information*. New York: Addison-Wesley.
Xue, C. C. L., Zhang, A. L., Lin, V., Costa, C. D. A., & Story, D. F. (2007). Complementary and alternative medicine use in Australia: A national population-based survey. *Journal of Alternative and Complementary Medicine, 13*, 643–650.

Chapter 9
The Psychological Roots of Health Promotion

Antonella Delle Fave

9.1 Introduction

The increasing attention paid by Western researchers, professionals, and policy makers to the active role and responsibility of the individuals in their own health management and disease prevention is deeply related to a variety of new challenges that postindustrial societies are facing today at the epidemiological, social, and economic levels. The relevance of this role is structurally embedded in the approach to health that has been characterizing Āyurveda throughout the millennia and across different social, historical, and natural contexts. Such a convergence between two very different medical systems is an interesting phenomenon that deserves deeper investigation, especially in the light of the potential of an integrated and synergistic perspective between the two systems in fostering human well-being and biopsychosocial health.

9.2 The Western Biopsychosocial Model and the Development of Health Psychology

The Western biomedical approach to disease is prominently focused on the biological and thus *objective* aspects of health conditions. While this approach gave great impulse to the advancements in the biomedical domain, its limitations were firstly highlighted by Engel (1977), who claimed the need for a biopsychosocial model, centered on the patient as a person with a cultural background and a subjective experience of health, disease, and quality of life (as highlighted in Chap. 2).

A. Delle Fave (✉)
Department of Pathophysiology and Transplantation, University of Milano, Milan, Italy
e-mail: antonella.dellefave@unimi.it

A. Morandi and A.N. Narayanan Nambi (eds.), *An Integrated View of Health and Well-being*, Cross-Cultural Advancements in Positive Psychology 5, DOI 10.1007/978-94-007-6689-1_9,

This claim was followed by a growing attention of researchers and policy makers to the individuals' *subjective* evaluation of their own health conditions (Levin and Browner 2005).

The relevance and the potentials of the biopsychosocial approach were promptly acknowledged by most international health agencies and institutions. Far from being a mere exercise of political correctness, this recognition stemmed out of the necessities imposed by the epidemiological profile that was increasingly characterizing human communities worldwide. The striking advancements in biomedical knowledge that took place during the twentieth century led to an epidemiological transition, particularly evident in postindustrial countries (Omran 1971; Barrett et al. 1998). The amazing development of pharmacology, the spreading of health-care facilities, improvements in diet, hygiene practices, and immunization campaigns led to a substantial reduction of infectious and acute diseases and to a relevant increase of life expectancy (as described in detail in Chap. 1). However, this positive trend was counterbalanced by the increase of chronic and degenerative diseases – prominently cardiovascular pathologies and cancer (WHO 2002) – partially related to aging but partially derived from massive urbanization and consequent lifestyle changes (Armelagos et al. 2005). The negative consequences of inappropriate dietary regimes, excessive workload, or inadequate physical exercise on cardiovascular and immune system functioning became increasingly evident.

In order to cope with these new challenges, specific effort was required to identify personal and social resources that could promote health and prevent disease onset or progression and complications, over and above medical interventions whose relevance was anyway limited, in case of chronic or degenerative diseases. To this purpose, in 1978 the division of health psychology was officially started by the American Psychological Association.

The impressive amount of constructs, models, and research studies that mushroomed within this domain in the following decades was grounded into a very clear evidence: two people sharing the same physical health conditions may largely differ as concerns their quality of life and overall level of well-being, on the basis of environmental and personal variables partially or totally independent of physical health conditions. This evidence brought to the attention of physicians, psychologists, and policy makers the necessity to systematically explore and operationalize the psychological and social components of health (Veenhoven 2002).

Most individuals develop effective strategies to cope with disease and related constraints that become prominently evident in conditions of chronic pathologies (Delle Fave 2010; Lazarus 2000). This effectiveness implies the availability of resources and positive dimensions in both the person and the environment, such as the ability to identify opportunities for action and skill development in daily life, the tendency to set and pursue goals, the detection and construction of meanings, and the support derived from positive social relations, community cohesion, and adequate health services (Joseph and Linley 2006; Kreuter 2000; Mytko and Knight 1999). A large amount of studies have been conducted to identify the mediating function on health of specific psychological features, such as perception of control (Fisher and Johnston 1996), coping style (Folkman and Greer 2000;

Galvin and Godfrey 2001; Pennebaker 1997; Stanton et al. 2000), self-efficacy (Bandura 1997, 2004; Kuijer and deRidder 2003), and resilience (Rolland and Walsh 2005). Other scholars have attempted to situate these psychological resources within broader constructs, trying to develop complex and integrated models of mental well-being.

9.2.1 Western Conceptualizations of Well-Being

Current conceptualizations of well-being in psychological terms involve two primary aspects: one related to pleasure and satisfaction derived from the fulfillment of needs and another related to the actualization of one's potentialities and pursuit of goals. They are subsumed under two broader frameworks – hedonia and eudaimonia (Ryan and Deci 2001; Delle Fave 2013a).

The hedonic approach moves from the core assumption that maximizing individual well-being is the highest human goal (Kahneman et al. 1999). The construct developed within this approach, subjective well-being (SWB, Diener 2000), includes an experiential component and an evaluative one. The experiential component consists in the presence of positive emotions and the absence of negative emotions (Fredrickson 2001). The cognitive evaluative component is the individual judgment on the level of satisfaction with one's life (Diener et al. 1985).

The eudaimonic view stems from Aristotle's concept of eudaimonia, described as the fulfillment of one's true nature, that includes both self-actualization and commitment to socially shared goals. According to Aristotle's conceptualization, well-being derives from the cultivation of personal resources and strengths through commitment to valuable activities and through the pursuit of both individual and collective goals. Within the eudaimonic approach in psychology, one of the more systematic conceptualizations was developed by Ryff (1989). It was labelled psychological well-being (PWB) and it comprises six dimensions: self-acceptance, positive relations, personal growth, purpose in life, mastery of environment, and autonomy. Keyes (1998) added to them five dimensions related to social well-being: social coherence, social actualization, social integration, social acceptance, and social contribution.

More recently, in the effort to develop a unified model of well-being, including both hedonic and eudaimonic components, Keyes (2003) revised the concept of mental health, defining it as a "syndrome" characterized by positive emotions, satisfaction with life, and optimal functioning at both the psychological and social levels. Individuals with a high level of mental health thrive and flourish, and this condition is relatively independent of their physical health conditions. On the opposite, the absence of mental health is characterized by languishing, stagnation, disengagement, and perception of an empty life. People who languish do not necessarily show symptoms of mental illness: however, they lack most of the symptoms of mental health. Flourishing and languishing represent two poles of the mental health continuum (MHC, Keyes 2005; Keyes et al. 2008), corresponding to health and absence of health, respectively (a thorough description of this model is provided in Chap. 1 of this volume).

This approach is consistent with the biopsychosocial model and with a definition of health (be it physical or mental) which does not simply consists in absence of disease, rather requiring the presence of "positive symptoms." Research has highlighted the positive impact of flourishing on physical health (Keyes 2007) and the usefulness of related tools and intervention strategies in the domain of clinical psychology (Fava and Ruini 2003, and Chap. 2 of this volume). In particular, a clinical approach focusing on inner resources and potentials, instead of weaknesses and deficits, can promote development and well-being in any situation, including objectively suboptimal conditions that cannot be substantially modified.

The conceptual relevance and practical usefulness of focusing on resources rather than on deficits were also embodied in the most recent revision of the international classifications of diseases and disabilities, which brought forth the new International Classification of Functioning (ICF; WHO 2001). ICF includes a marked shift in terminology, from pathology and constraints (impairments, disabilities, handicaps) to health and resources (functioning), from the consequences of disease to the components of health. ICF aims at investigating what people with different health conditions actually *can do* in their daily life and in their social context, emphasizing the active interaction of the person with the environment, in terms of physical resource mobilization, daily activity performance, and social participation. Far from being a pure linguistic convention, a relevant conceptual change underlies this shift from disease to functioning, leading to the evaluation of health conditions from a constructive and substantially positive perspective.

More recently, Western researchers have been paying growing attention to a specific and previously overlooked concept: well-being as harmony and balance, at both the individual and the social level. From a need-focused perspective, Sirgy and Wu (2009) defined balance as a state "reflecting satisfaction or fulfillment in several important domains with little or no negative affect in other domains" (p. 185), prominently referring to the satisfaction of needs and expectations in crucial life areas such as family, work, and health. Another study (Wu 2009) highlighted that in order to maintain high levels of life satisfaction humans tend to attribute higher importance to the life domains characterized by a low discrepancy between need perception and need fulfillment.

From a state-focused perspective, a recent study conducted in seven Western countries (Delle Fave et al. 2011a) highlighted that when asked to define happiness, lay people prominently refer to inner harmony and balance, describing it as inner peace, self-acceptance, serenity, and as a condition of equipoise and evenness. Ryan et al. (2008) identified the prominent outcome of a eudaimonically lived existence with a feeling of inner harmony and connectedness with the environment leading to self-transcendence.

By the way, the relevance of inner balance to a good life is not new in the Western tradition (Delle Fave 2013b): Plato included harmony in his definition of the just man; Aristotle invited to seek "the intermediate," avoiding any excess or deficiency in behaviors, attitudes, beliefs, and expectations; the Stoics pursued the ideal of evenness of judgment and detachment; and Epicurus focused on ataraxia, the attainment of balance and equipoise in both positive and negative situations. The concept of inner harmony is also shared by all Asian philosophical traditions, in which it was formalized in a much more systematic and effective way, as described with regard to Āyurveda in the following pages.

9.2.2 *The Active Role of the Person in Health Management*

One of the prominent concerns shared by researchers and practitioners in the health domain is the necessity to make people aware of their own active role in preserving health and in adaptively managing disease. In the last three decades, several models were developed, in order to identify the environmental and psychological mechanisms underlying health-related behaviors, with the aim of promoting the agency and responsibility of individuals in promoting and maximizing their own health and well-being.

The most effective models focus on the human capacity for intentional goal setting and its relevance to the pursuit of health behaviors, especially when changes in lifestyle and behavior are required in order to maintain or retrieve health (smoke or alcohol abuse, inappropriate diet, risk exposure, dysfunctional daily habits). Prochaska and DiClemente (1984) proposed a dynamic model, the *Transtheoretical Model of Change*, that has been extensively applied in prevention and healthcare programs (Cropley et al. 2003; Prochaska et al. 1994; Spencer et al. 2002). The model is articulated in five stages: individuals must first become aware of their health problems and goals (the contemplation stage) and then develop an intentional strategy to attain them, put it into practice, and actively contribute to the maintenance of the achieved results, which can also imply to cope with possible relapses.

The intentional change process depicted in Prochaska and DiClemente's model can take place by virtue of the mobilization of psychological and social resources. Among them, self-efficacy (Bandura 1977) is prominent. Self-efficacy can be defined as the level of competence an individual perceives in facing a specific situation. It facilitates the intentional mobilization of personal resources and skills in the long term. Self-efficacious people are relatively unaffected by failures, and they show high levels of perseverance in pursuing their goals. Self-efficacy has proved to be useful in coping with adverse health conditions, since highly self-efficacious people face negative life events actively, perceiving themselves as directly responsible for the outcome. Also in situations characterized by low controllability – such as permanent disabilities or the terminal stage of a disease – self-efficacious individuals are advantaged, in that their perception of an adequate level of competence allows them to develop effective coping strategies, a good management of emotions, and the capacity to set and attain realistic goals (Merluzzi and Sanchez 1997; Hurley and Shea 1992).

Other researchers have confirmed the role of intentional processing of information in pursuing health goals (see, e.g., Gollwitzer and Oettingen 1998). Broadly speaking, these models emphasize the importance of agency, a core construct in psychology that has been conceptualized in various ways (for an overview, see

Bassi et al. 2010). According to Bandura (1997), the sense of agency emerges from intentional behavior and high self-efficacy beliefs. From a motivational and developmental perspective, Deci and Ryan (2000) refer human agency to motivated behaviors that emanate from one's integrated self. To be agentic is to be self-determined and thus to be autonomous form environmental conditionings. The prototypical activity from which agency emerges as an integrated process is the intrinsically motivated behavior, performed when individuals perceive themselves free from environmental demands and constraints. Agency is of paramount importance for the patients' participation in any health-related process, ranging from adherence to treatments to all the stages of prevention (Gregor et al. 2006; Kipling et al. 2005; Sheldon et al. 2003). Agency as a condition of shared power and responsibility is one of the five pillars of the patient-centered model of relationship, in which the physician encourages patients' active participation and decision-making in the selection of their treatment and in the long-term monitoring of their disease course (Mead and Bower 2000; Mead et al. 2002).

From a broader and eudaimonic perspective, the economist Amartya Sen (1992) defined the sense of agency as the property according to which individuals undertake relevant and meaningful actions taking into account the relation between the person, the social context, and other people's needs. This approach emphasizes the mobilization and implementation of personal skills and resources, the cultivation of social competencies and interpersonal relations, and the pursuit of aims and activities which are meaningful for the individual and for the society. Research studies have highlighted that agency and responsibility as eudaimonic resources are actually mobilized in stressful situations. At the community level, natural disasters are often opportunities to strengthen social ties and to promote solidarity: for example, a decrease in the number of psychiatric hospitalizations, drug use, and police reports was detected following a devastating tornado (Quarantelli 1985). At the individual level, people are able to identify the positive consequences of a negative event such as the onset of a disease (Sodergren and Hyland 2000). Most often, these consequences refer to developmental changes that contribute to make the individual a better person, more aware of own strengths and weaknesses, less vulnerable to daily stressors, more open to relationships, and more focused on meaningful goals and priorities.

The crucial importance of agency in health and well-being promotion is not surprising. The most recent conceptualizations of human development have highlighted the process of *daily psychological selection* (Csikszentmihalyi and Massimini 1985), through which individuals differentially replicate subsets of the biological and cultural information available to them in their daily environment, thus actively contributing to its survival and changes (Massimini and Delle Fave 2000). Psychological selection results from the person's preferential investment of attention and resources on a limited amount of the environmental opportunities for action and engagement. In particular, when daily activities are perceived as sources of well-being and positive experiences, their preferential cultivation provides the individual with increasingly complex competences and skills, fostering personal growth and development (Delle Fave and Massimini 2005). Several cross-cultural studies (summarized in Delle Fave et al. 2011b) showed that two core elements play a key role in guiding psychological selection. The first one is the association of specific activities with optimal experience, or flow (Csikszentmihalyi 1975/2000), characterized by engagement, skill investment, involvement, and enjoyment. The second component is the long-term meaning individuals attribute to the daily activities available to them (Delle Fave 2009; Schlegel et al. 2011). Through the attribution of meaning to specific life activities and domains, individuals pursue goals they deem as relevant, as well as consistent with social values and others' needs.

Except for extreme conditions, each person usually has a more or less wide range of activities at their disposal, on which to perform an active psychological selection (Delle Fave and Massimini 2004). However, it is important to consider that the evolution trend supported by this process does not necessarily lead to well-being or higher quality of life. The ultimate result depends upon the type of activities and goals individuals decide to pursue. In order to bring developmentally positive effects, psychological selection has to promote internal order and integration of the individual and at the same time constructive information exchange with the environment, the latter comprising social integration as well as commitment to the improvement of the culture and of the quality of life of the other community members (Delle Fave 2007). These prerequisites are consistent with the conceptualization of human beings as complex living systems, described in Chap. 10 of this volume.

Based on the WHO definition of health as a global condition of well-being that includes biological, psychological, and social components, the active and long-term involvement of each individual in preserving and improving it implies the development of skills and competences, meanings and goals, behaviors, and relationships that selectively allow for a positive health management. Far from being a simple task, this endeavor requires high self-efficacy beliefs and commitment to long-term goals, adaptive preferential selection of the environmental information, effective coping strategies in the face of challenges and stressors, positive interpersonal relationships, and the ability to constructively interact with the environment (Cortinovis et al. 2011; Ryff and Singer 2008). According to the Western psychological view, all these competences and resources are not innate and genetically based features, but they can be learned through commitment and practice. They can be therefore cultivated by any individual. As described in the following sections, these features are consistent with the Ayurvedic assumptions concerning healthy behaviors and lifestyle.

9.3 Life, Health, and Well-Being in Āyurveda

According to the *Sāṃkhya* conceptualization (referred to in Chap. 3), which is followed by most Āyurveda scholars, the universe stemmed from the interaction between two eternal and unmanifest principles: *puruṣa* (conscious and passive) and *Prakṛti* (the dynamic and unconscious source of all manifestations). This interaction led to the manifestation and differentiation of all living entities, *starting* from *mahat* (the universal order) and *ahaṃkāra* (the individual identity). *Ahaṃkāra* has three different qualities (*guṇa*): *sattva* (balance, equilibrium, clarity), *rajas* (dynamism), and *tamas* (inertia). The interaction between *sattva* and *rajas* produces eleven *indriyas* (sense and motor organs) as well as *manas* (the mind, coordinating the senses' activity). *Tamas* and *rajas* combine to produce five *tanmātrās* (primordial units of perceivable matter), which in their turn produce the five *mahabhutas* (great elements): *ākash* (ether), *vāyu (air), tejas (fire), ap (water),* and *pṛthvi (earth*), manifest aggregates of matter. From these *mahabhutas* the entire material world is made up (Dash and Junius 1983). Both unmanifest principles – eternal consciousness and the source of nature – are thus embodied in each living being. The individual soul or self (*ātman*), eternal and unchangeable, is ontologically identical to the universal consciousness principle (also defined *Brahman*). *Ātman* is present in every living being, and after the death of the body, it migrates in another being, carrying the impressions (*saṃskāra*) of the previous lives.

Consistently with this perspective, the great Āyurveda scholar Ćaraka defines life – *Ayus* – as composed by mind (*manas*), self (*ātman*), and body (*sarira*) (Ćaraka Saṃhitā, Sūtra Sthāna: 1, 46–47 in Sharma and Baghwan Dash 1998). Within the Ayurvedic mind-body system, the *ātman* plays the role of witness, taking no active part in the interaction of the individual with the environment. The *ātman* is therefore pure consciousness, and in essence it is happiness and bliss, *ananda*. However, humans can hardly experience this condition due to a set of sheaths (*kosha*) covering this core essence. The *kosha* are thoroughly described in Chap. 2, *Brahmānanda Valli* of the Taittiriya Upanishad (Swami Chinmayananda 1992). The most external one is *annamaykosha*, the physical body strictly related to food (*anna*), followed by *prānamayakosha* (the vital energy, connected to breath), *manomayakosha* (the mental sheath, in which the basic psychological functions related to perception and memory take place), and *vijnānamayakosha* (the intelligence sheath, characterized by discernment, discrimination, and determination). The core sheath, *ānandamayakosha*, is the sheath of bliss, the abode of *ātman*: at this level "the individual is free from the notions of egoism and sense of agency, the characteristic features of *manomaya* and *vijanamaya* respectively" (Kuppuswami 1985, p. 20).

Individuals however differ according to the prominence they give to different *kosha*, by relating their essential identity to a particular set of functions and dimensions. The majority of people tend to identify themselves with the first three *kosha*, thus being conditioned by positive and negative emotions, attachment to external objects, and mind fluctuations (Kiran Kumar 2006). This is prominently due to the fact that the ceaseless contact with external and internal stimuli makes the mind wander like a "restless monkey" across different feelings, thoughts, and experiences. This dependency of the individual on pleasure/pain feelings and subsequent attraction/repulsion behaviors originates from the interaction of the mind with environmental objects or inner triggers. It represents the ultimate cause of suffering in that the transient nature of pleasure generates further desire, craving, and longing for the associated objects, while pain directly produces suffering. This view of mind is substantially shared by all the Indian philosophical systems (Kiran Kumar 2003). Since the individual is entrapped into this web of unstable and ultimately distressing experience fluctuations within the *manomayakosha*, human evolution is considered as the progressive actualization of higher levels of consciousness towards the experience of *ānanda,* in which the knower, the object of knowledge, and the act of knowing merge into a single entity. The ultimate goal of human beings is to get rid of the constraints of sensory attractions and mind fluctuations and to identify with the state of perfect bliss which characterizes *ātman*.

In the Kena Upanishad, this concept is beautifully synthesized as follows:

> If one knows That *Brahman* here, in this world, then the true end of all human aspirations is gained. If one knows not That here, great is the destruction. The wise, seeing the one *Ātman* in all beings, rise from sense-life and become immortal. (Kena Upanishad: 2, 5 in Swami Chinmayananda 1952)

The concept of *purushārtha*, goals of human existence, is particularly relevant to this purpose. Depending on one's stage of psychological development, people may pursue desires (*kāma*), wealth (*artha*), personal and collective values (*dharma*), and liberation (*mokṣa*). The pursuit of desires and wealth to the exclusion of pursuit of values and of liberation is however a sign of lower level of evolution.

Individuals widely differ in their needs and aspirations; some of them are purely hedonistic, a few are spiritual in nature, while the vast majority falls in between. In the light of this evidence, in the Indian culture, a social framework and ground rules were developed to promote good life by giving equal importance to *dharma, artha*, and *kāma* (Kiran Kumar 2004):

> the correct position is that the good of man consists of the harmonious co-ordination of the three. (Manu, II: 224; in Banerjee 1980)

The relative importance of each of the three "lower" human goals clearly emerges in the writing of Āyurveda scholars such as Ćaraka and Vagbhata, who relate it to health:

> So a wise person ... should strive for discarding the harmful or unwholesome regimens and adopt the wholesome ones in regard to *dharma, artha*, and *kāma*, for no happiness or unhappiness can occur in this world without these three elements. (Ćaraka Saṃhitā, Sūtra Sthāna: 11,46 in Sharma and Baghwan Dash 1998)
>
> Person desiderous of (long) life which is the means for achieving *dharma, artha,* and *sukha* should repose utmost faith in the teachings of Āyurveda. (Aṣṭāṅga Hṛdaya, Sūtra Sthāna: 1,2 in Srikantha Murthy 2007)

9.3.1 Health and Well-Being as Balance

If we try to draw a comparison with the Western conceptualizations of well-being described in the previous sections, the hedonic approach is more related to *kāma* and to *artha,* while *dharma* with its different individual and social connotations encompasses the concept of eudaimonia (Kiran Kumar 2003). Western theories of happiness and well-being however limit their exploration and conceptualization to the first three goals without considering the last one, *mokṣa*. On the opposite, in the Indian thought, the ideal well-being is understood as an outcome of the expansion of consciousness and realization of a transcendent self whose very nature is *ānanda*. Its manifestation is obstructed by the dullness of our mental faculties, derived from the prominent investment of psychological resources on inner or external sources of pleasure and pain, which – as discussed above – generates attachment and ultimately suffering. The increasing balance in the mental functioning (i.e., the prominence of their *sattva* quality on *tamas* and *rajas)* facilitates the experience of *ānanda*. Patanjali's Yoga Sūtras specifically describe the process leading to liberation through the experience of identification with the *ātman*, as well as the eight steps required to attain it (Feuerstein 1998). In the Bhagavad Gitā, all these concepts are made accessible to a broader audience and applicable to ordinary people's life. In particular, the core concept of this scripture is the pursuit of nonattachment (*anāsakti*), a condition of mental balance and equanimity in dealing with life events without being emotionally affected by their positive or negative features and consequences (Swami Chinmayananda 1975). The ideal of *anāsakti* embodies spiritual growth as well as action orientation. To be detached does not mean to withdraw from life demands and duties. Rather it implies to perform any action with dispassion, without concerns for failure or success, loss or gains (Pande and Naidu 1992):

> A courageous man is not one who does heroic acts but the one who is tranquil in mind under any circumstances of agitation. (Kalidas, quoted by Thirumulpadu 2010, p. 55)

Therefore, well-being and good life can be achieved through surrendering rather than controlling and holding on; minimization, restraint, and detachment from need fulfillment are more effective in promoting well-being than maximization, indulgence, and striving for need fulfillment (Kiran Kumar 2004).

The focus on balance in mind and behavior as the basic prerequisite for health and well-being is repeatedly stated by all the major scholars of Āyurveda with reference to body, mind, and behavior:

> Disease is disequilibrium of the *dhātu* Health is equilibrium of *dhātu*. Health is known as pleasure. Disease is known as pain. (Ćaraka Saṃhitā, Sūtra Sthāna: 9,4 in Sharma and Baghwan Dash 1998)

In this quotation, *dhātu* refers to the structural constituents of the body that can be loosely explained as tissues (a more detailed description of *dhātu* is provided in Chap. 10). *Ćaraka* attributed the state of perfect health/balance to the ancestors living in the age of perfection, *kritayuga*, during which humans were in direct contact with the divine, following the laws of dharma and a virtuous lifestyle (Ćaraka Saṃhitā, VimanaSthāna 3:24–25, in Sharma and Baghwan Dash 1998).

An effective synthesis of this interpretation of health can be found in *Suśruta Saṃhitā*, where the term used for health is *swasthya*, that means "to be established (*Sthya*) in oneself (*Swa*)." According to *Suśruta* (Suśruta Saṃhitā, Sūtra Sthāna: 15, in Kaviraj Kunjalal Bhishagratna 1911), a person is established in oneself when her physiological functions and structures are in a state of equilibrium, together with contentment of mind, discriminative intellect, and senses.

9.3.2 *Prakṛti and Health*

At the psychophysical level, the natural state of balance was formalized in terms of a key concept in Āyurveda: three principles known as doṣa – *vāta, pitta*, and *kapha*. They are not thought of as specifically physiological but rather as principles that emerge in the manifestation of the individual as a complex system (as described in Chaps. 4 and 10). They derive from the combination of the five *Mahabhutas*: *vāta* is prominently constituted of *vayu* and *ākash*; *pitta* of *tejas* and *ap*; and *kapha* of *ap* and *pṛthvi*. Together with the seven tissues and the waste products, they represent "the roots of the body always" (Aṣṭāṅga Hṛdaya, Sūtra Sthāna: 11, 1, in Srikantha Murthy 2007).

The three *doṣa* as functional principles subsume all the strategic activities of human life, at both the physical and mental levels (Subramanya Sastri 2009, and Chap. 4 in this volume). More specifically, from a functional perspective, *vāta* is expressed in the body and mind movements, such as blood flow, peristalsis, breathing, changes and fluctuations in perception and thought, sensory activities, and generation of ideas. *Vāta* controls *pitta* and *kapha* and is usually the first cause of disease. When in excess, at the psychological level, it leads to anxiety, insomnia, and mood instability, while at the physical level, it generates increase in degenerative processes, irregularity of system functions, and loss in tissue mass and compactness. *Pitta* is manifest in the transformation processes that take place in the mind and body, such as food digestion, hormone regulation, the processing and elaboration of sensorial information, and the cognitive ability of discriminating and discerning. *Pitta* must be kept in balance, too, since its excess may lead at the psychological level to anger, aggressiveness, and competitiveness and at the physical level to acceleration of metabolic processes and inflammatory pathologies. *Kapha*, whose constituents are water and earth, is reflected in the body cohesion and stability. It is related to physical strength and vigor, and it promotes immunity and resilience to external injuries. It is associated with memory strength and emotional stability; with calmness, forgiveness, and love; and with loyalty and patience. Too much *kapha* leads to lethargy and drowsiness and to feelings of attachment, greed, and envy at the psychological level; at the physical level, it leads to weight increase, water retention, and a global reduction in metabolic processes.

The conceptualization of the *doṣa* is rooted into in the Vedic scriptures. In Prasna Upanishad, for example, there is a detailed description of the *vāta* subcomponent, called *subdoṣa*, starting from *prana* as the life principle (Swami Chinmayananda 1954). The three *doṣa* pervade the entire being encompassing the body, emotions, and mind, and according to their relative proportions, they determine the constitutional type of the individual, or *Prakṛti* (Ćaraka Saṃhitā, Sūtra Sthāna: 30,25, and Aṣṭāṅga Hṛdaya, ŚārīraSthāna*:* 3, 83 in Srikantha Murthy 2007).

In Sanskrit *Prakṛti* means "the natural condition or state of anything, of nature, of a natural form," the root *kri* meaning "to make," and the prefix *pra* "forward, forth, in front, onward." Thus, it evokes notions of first cause or first action. As a matter of fact, individuals with different *Prakṛti* differ from one another in their body structure and functioning, capacity for immunity from disease, emotional responses, and psychological characteristics.

The literature on *doṣa* and *Prakṛti* is extremely vast, and it was substantially expanded by the recent scientific evidence derived from studies focusing on their genetic bases (Juyal et al. 2012; Patwardhan and Bodeker 2008; Prasher et al. 2008). For the sake of synthesis and to the purposes of this chapter, only the description of the three basic typologies of *Prakṛti*, related to the predominance of one *doṣa* over the other two, will be reported here. To this purpose, the description provided by *Ćaraka* was selected, since further developments added very little to such an astonishingly detailed and precise classification (Ćaraka Saṃhitā, VimanaSthāna 8: 96–98 in Sharma and Baghwan Dash 1998):

> *Vāta* is ununctuous, light, mobile, abundant in quantity, swift, cold, rough and non-slime. Various manifestations due to these attributes of *vāta* in human body having *vātala* type of constitution are ununctuousness, emaciation and dwarfness of the body, longdrawn, low, broken, obstructed and hoarse voice, and sleeplessness; light and inconsistent gait, activities, diet and movement; unstable joints, eyes, eye brows, jaws, lips, tongue, head, shoulder, hands and legs; talkativeness, abundance in tendons and veins; quickness in initiating actions, in getting irritated and in the onset of morbid manifestations, quickness in affliction with fear, likes and dislikes, in understanding and forgetting things; intolerance to cold, affliction with cold, shivering and stiffness; coarseness in the hair of the head, face and other parts of the body, nails, teeth, face, hands and feet; cracking of the limbs and organs, cracking sounds in joints when they move. By virtue of the above mentioned qualities, persons having *vātala*[1] type of constitution mostly have lesser quantity of strength, life span, progeny, accessories of life and wealth.
>
> *Pitta* is hot, sharp, liquid, of fleshy smell, sour and pungent. Various manifestations due to these attributes in the human body having *pittala* type of constitution are intolerance for of hot things, hot face, tender and clear body, freckles, black moles, pimples, excessive hunger and thirst, quick advent of wrinkles, greying of hair and baldness, presence of soft and brown hair in the face, head, and other parts of the body; demonstration of sharp physical strength, strong digestive power, intake of food and drink in large quantity, inability to face difficult situations and glutton habits; looseness and softness of joints and muscles, excess sweat, urine and feces; putrid smell of axilla, mouth, head and body; insufficiency of semen, sexual desire and procreation. By virtue of the above mentioned qualities the person having *pittala*[2] type of constitution is endowed with moderate strength, life-span, spiritual and materialistic knowledge, understanding, wealth, and the accessories of life.
>
> *Kapha* is unctuous, smooth, soft, sweet, firm, dense, slow, stable, heavy, cold, viscous, and clear. The various manifestations in the human body having *śleṣmala*[3] type of constitution are unctuous and smooth organs; pleasing appearance, tenderness and clarity of complexion; abundant semen, desire for sex-act and number of progeny; firmness, compactness and stability of the body; plumpness and roundedness of all organs; slowness in action, intake of food and movement; slowness in initiating action, getting irritated and morbid manifestations; non slippery and stable gait with the entire sole of the feet pressing against the earth; little hunger, thirst, heat, and perspiration; firmness and compactness in joints; happiness in the look and face; happiness and softness of complexion and voice. By virtue of the above mentioned qualities, a person having *śleṣmala* type of constitution is endowed with the excellence of strength, wealth, knowledge, energy, peace, and longevity.

[1] in which *vata* prevails.

[2] in which *pitta* prevails.

[3] in which *kapha*, also called *śleṣma*, prevails.

9.3.3 *Vikṛti and Disease: The Role of Mind*

The healthy *Prakṛti* is a state of a dynamic equilibrium of *doṣa, dhātu, mala* (waste products), and *agni* (the principle of transformation and assimilation power); it shows an intrinsic order that is disturbed by aggravation or decrease in the proportion of its constitutive *doṣa* (*vikṛti*), which affect the body and mind functioning. It is important however to consider that disease is only proximally due to *doṣa* imbalance. The primary causes of this imbalance have to be identified at the mental level. The interaction between the individual and environment occurs through three channels, namely, *prajna* (or *buddhi*, the intellective *guṇa* or quality of the mind, as defined by the *Nyāya Vaiśeṣika* system and endorsed by Āyurveda scholars, e.g., Ćaraka Saṃhitā, ŚārīraSthāna: 1, 49 in Sharma and Baghwan Dash 1998), *indriyas* (the senses), and *kala* (the seasons and nature rhythms). The deviations of *prajna, indriyas,* or *kala* from their balanced state are the original sources of diseases, whose prominent early symptom will be vitiation of *doṣa* (Ćaraka Saṃhitā: Sūtra Sthāna: 20, 5; ŚārīraSthāna: 1, 198–132 in Sharma and Baghwan Dash 1998).

In particular, *prajnaparādha* refers to wrong understanding and decision-making, wrong discernment, and going against knowledge. *Asatmyendriyārthasamyoga* refers to wrong contact of the sense organs with the environmental stimuli, through their abuse, misuse, or nonuse; and *kala pariṇāma* refers to the inability or inattention of the person to get tuned with the changing cycles of nature (see Chap. 5 for a more detailed description of the factors contributing to imbalance and health alterations). These errors lead to unwholesome behavior and thus generate *doṣa* imbalance and disease. *Ćaraka* however highlights that

> Neither the sense organs nor their objects alone can bring about happiness or miseries. The latter are in fact caused by the fourfold combination (proper use, wrong use, excessive use, non use). Even if there are sense organs and their objects present, there would be no disease, nor any happiness unless the fourfold combination is involved. (Ćaraka Saṃhitā, ŚārīraSthāna : 1, 130–131 in Sharma and Baghwan Dash 1998)

It is therefore clear that since *manas*, the mind, coordinates and influences the actions and contacts of the sense organs, on the one side, and the knowledge and discrimination faculties of the intellect, or *buddhi*, on the other side, a perturbed mind represents the basic source of ill-being and disease.

More specifically, a relevant role in disease onset is played by the three mental *guṇa*: *sattva*, *rajas*, and *tamas,* which represent the principle of equilibrium, dynamism, and inertia, respectively. *Tamas* is responsible for dullness, retardation, and depression. *Rajas* is responsible for energy and action. *Sattva* is responsible for balance, harmony, and awareness. The higher the proportion of *sattva* compared to the other two *guṇa*, the more is the mind balanced, allowing for the achievement of a closer identification with the *ātman,* beyond the emotional fluctuations generated by the attachment to the sense objects.

These three *maha guṇa*, as described above and analyzed with greater details in Chaps. 3, 4, and 10, are the substantial qualities that constitute the eternal and active principle of *Prakṛti*. The original interaction between *Prakṛti* and *puruṣa* generates an imbalance among the three *maha guṇa,* leading to the development of the manifest reality. *Maha guṇa* are thus constituents of the whole reality, including human beings. All the three *guṇa* are present in all the individuals, regardless of their *doṣa Prakṛti,* and they are involved in the deviations from the correct functioning of *prajna, indriyas,* or *kala* perception, reported above as main causes of imbalance in the *doṣa.* At the mental level, individuals can be differentiated as *sāttvic, rājasic,* and *tāmasic* depending on the preponderance of one *guṇa* over the other two. Following the synthetic description provided by Kiran Kumar (2003), a *sāttvic* person shows discriminative intellect: self-control, serenity and equipoise, and freedom from attachment and from the fruits of action. A *rājasic* person is driven into action by passion; has desires, strong likes, and dislikes; and lacks clear discrimination. A *tāmasic* person is depressed, lethargic, negligent, undisciplined, arrogant, ignorant, and dull. The three *guṇa,* as the qualities of the mind, are responsible for the individual differences in mood and attitudes.

The interplay between *guṇa* and *doṣa* is clarified by Ćaraka:

> Mental faculty is of three types—*Sattva, Rajas* and *Tamas.* The *Sattva* is said as devoid of defects due to having beneficial fraction whereas *Rajas* and *Tamas* are defective because of the fractions of agitation and ignorance respectively. Out of these three types of psyche, each one has got innumerable sub-divisions due to relative degrees and variations in interaction of psyche and body according to species. (Ćaraka Saṃhitā, ŚārīraSthāna: 4, 36 in Sharma and Baghwan Dash 1998)

Recently, Frawley (2004) has stressed the importance to evaluate *doṣa* and *guṇa* in their interplay, in order to cover all the biological, psychological, and spiritual implications for well-being of their balance or imbalance. Western scholars are presently exploring the scientific evidence and role of *doṣa* at the biological and physiological levels and in different species (Hankey 2010).

9.4 The Psychological Roots of Health in Āyurveda and in the Biopsychosocial Model: Convergences and Divergences

The brief excursus provided in the previous pages on the role of the individual mind in health promotion and disease prevention in Western medicine and in Āyurveda allows for some comparative considerations that are aimed to highlight commonalities and differences between the two approaches.

9.4.1 Health as a Multifaceted Construct

Both Āyurveda and the biopsychosocial model acknowledge the complexity of health as a multifaceted outcome resulting from the interplay of several systems. As concerns the conceptual background, however, Āyurveda situates individual health within a unitary framework in which morphophysiological, psychological, and behavioral features are taken into account all together and related to a whole set of environmental dimensions that range from seasonal cycles to social relationships, from collective *dharma* to cosmic influences. The Western biopsychosocial model, though attempting to provide an interconnected view of the three different systems involved in the evaluation of health, does not aim to bring them together into a unified conceptualization. In particular, the role of the psychological resources and potentials of the person in dealing with health and disease (the "psycho") has become specific objects of investigation of health psychology, a new additional branch of the discipline, separated and autonomous from medicine (the "bio") and from sociology and economics (the "social"). This approach is consistent with the tendency towards compartmentalization typical of Western science.

An interesting convergence between Āyurveda and the Western conception of well-being at both the psychological and overall health levels concerns the importance of balance, a dimension only recently rediscovered in Western psychology.

9.4.2 Disease Onset

In Āyurveda the interplay between the mind and the body is formalized in hierarchical terms, being grounded in a cosmological view in which subtler entities are superior to grosser entities: this is reflected in the five *kosha* representation and in the classification of the three substantial causes of health and disease, all being located at the level of *manas* – either in its connections with the sense organs and related behaviors or with the discrimination and intellectual functions. This approach clearly situates the prominent responsibility for health preservation in the person as a psychic entity. In the Western approach, the relationships between biological and psychological features are not hierarchically defined, although a tendency towards biological reductionism cannot be denied: when speaking about health, Western medicine usually refers to physical health. Causes of disease are usually identified in external agents or in altered conditions of the body functions, and their effects are evaluated prominently at the physical level. Even in case of psychiatric disorders, the greatest efforts are put in detecting their biological and anatomo-physiological origins or correlates. This substantial difference is surely due to the different conceptualization of etiology and pathogenesis in the two medical systems: doṣa imbalance (*sañcaya*) is the first stage of pathogenesis in Āyurveda, and treatment should take place at this stage, where balance can be easily retrieved. The organ-related manifestation of disease (*vyadhi vyakti*) represents the fifth stage that takes place long time after the occurrence of *doṣa* imbalance and that is much more difficult to treat. Within the Western model of medicine, people usually consult the physician only when a manifest disease is present, ignoring the previous signals of imbalance or treating them with generic and palliative medicaments. This neglect would be classified in Āyurveda as *prajnaparadha.* The impressive increase in lifestyle-related diseases in postindustrial countries has recently given impulse to a growing awareness of the importance of preventive healthy behaviors, thus calling into play individual responsibility, agency, and psychological selection. As outlined in the previous pages, various intervention models have been developed to help people leave unhealthy habits or adopt healthy ones through the mobilization of psychological resources. However, in spite of such an overwhelming research evidence of the potentials of prevention, most people still wait for the disease manifestation at the organ level before seriously undertaking these efforts.

9.4.3 Health Management

In Āyurveda, the various manifestations of health and disease substantially depend on the individual *Prakṛti*. As a consequence, remedies, treatments, and preventive measures must be personalized according to the constitution of the single individual, based on the proportion of *guṇa* and *doṣa*. Insomnia in a *vātala* person should be treated differently from insomnia in a *ślesmala* one, through the prescription of *Prakṛti*-specific medicaments, diet, and changes in lifestyle. The constructs and theories developed within Western health psychology are instead assumed as universally valid for any individual, based on the Western view of psychological functioning as a system of functions and mechanisms working in the same way across individuals. From this perspective, all people are supposed to be able to mobilize the same inner resources and to adopt the same prevention strategies when facing health problems. In so doing, health psychology entails the risk of neglecting not only psychological differences but also geographical and cultural variations. Specific behaviors, activities, or habits do not necessarily have the same meaning or function in different cultures: therefore, we should not expect them to have an invariant relation to well-being or health (Deci and Ryan 2000). For example, physical training – largely popular in Western countries – can become problematic in a social context characterized by a different emphasis on fitness and body image, a different gender role pattern, or a different climate. Dietary regimens cannot ignore the food habits and related social norms of the patients. Standardization of treatments at both the physical and psychological levels is one of the major weaknesses of the Western approach to health.

9.4.4 The Self

In Āyurveda, the mind is contextualized into an articulated philosophical and cosmological view, in which the dimension of transcendence plays a pivotal role. As briefly outlined in the previous pages, the human being is constituted by the tripod of body, mind, and *ātman*, the self, ontologically identical to *Brahman,* the all pervading eternal principle of reality, without attributes and dimensions. Among the goals that individuals pursue in their life, the highest one is *mokṣa*, the liberation from the attachment to passions and sense objects, that is grounded in the prominence of *sattva* among the mental *guṇa* and in the progressive development of the person towards the innermost layer of the individuality, the *ānandamayakosha*. In this lies the true *swāsthya*, health and well-being (Kiran Kumar 2006). Āyurveda itself as a knowledge system developed from the spiritual tradition of the Veda, Sākhya, and Yoga Sutras. The spiritual component is thus seen as a substantial constituent of the person's health. In the Western biopsychosocial approach, spirituality and religion have been indeed object of research, and several epidemiological studies have emphasized the benefits of spirituality and religiosity on health. A positive correlation was detected between religious practice and health (Larson et al. 1989; McCullough et al. 1999). This has been ascribed to various factors: most religious systems prescribe healthy lifestyles and food habits; prayer and meditation foster psychophysical relaxation; practicing religion promotes social support through more stable family ties and the participation to community rituals; and religiosity provides meanings and hope and fosters a more active acceptance of negative events (Jenkins and Pargament 1995; Park and Folkman 1997; McClain et al. 2003). However, the religious/spiritual dimension is considered as a private issue, and it is not included per se in any model of health and well-being, rather representing one of the psychological resources available to the individual when facing health problems.

9.5 Concluding Remarks

The synthetic outline provided in the previous pages has clearly highlighted a convergent pathway between Western science and Āyurveda in the evaluation of the individuals as primary and responsible agents of their own health. The psychological dimensions, resources, and processes identified by health psychology are consistent with the view provided in the classical texts of Āyurveda. Nevertheless, the two approaches show major differences, especially as concerns the relevance attributed to the transcendent dimension, the recognition of early symptoms, and the typological distinction of the individuals based on their *doṣa* proportion. While the spiritual aspects are grounded into traditions and cultural beliefs that cannot be generalized, the Ayurvedic warning about the education to prevention, through a greater awareness of one's own healthy or unhealthy behaviors, food habits, and lifestyle, could be usefully integrated in the Western knowledge. Similarly, more attention should be attributed to the person's psychophysical peculiarities, overcoming the tendency to standardize treatments and behavioral guidelines. The growing concern for health and well-being can find effective suggestions in the teaching of the ancient Indian scholars.

References

Armelagos, G., Brown, P., & Turner, B. (2005). Evolutionary, historical and political economic perspectives on health and disease. *Social Science & Medicine, 61*, 755–765.

Bandura, A. (1977). Self-efficacy: Toward a unifying theory of behavioural change. *Psychological Review, 84*, 191–215.

Bandura, A. (1997). *Self-efficacy: The exercise of control*. New York: Freeman.
Bandura, A. (2004). Health promotion by social cognitive means. *Health Education & Behavior, 31*, 143–164.
Banerjee, N. V. (1980). *Studies in the Dharmasastra of Manu*. New Delhi: Munshiram Manoharlal.
Barrett, R., Kuzawa, C., Mcdade, T., & Armelagos, G. (1998). Emerging infectious disease and the third epidemiological transition. In W. Durham (Ed.), *Annual review of anthropology* (pp. 247–271). Palo Alto: Annual Reviews Inc.
Bassi, M., Sartori, R., & Delle Fave, A. (2010). The monitoring of experience and agency in daily life: A study with Italian adolescents. In M. Balconi (Ed.), *Neuropsychology of the sense of agency. From consciousness to action* (pp. 81–105). Milan: Springer.
Bhishagratna, K. K. (1911). *The Suśruta Saṃhitā* (English translation). Calcutta: K.K. Bhishagratna.
Cortinovis, I., Luraschi, E., Intini, S., Sessa, M., & Delle Fave, A. (2011). The daily experience of people with achondroplasia. *Applied Psychology: Health and Well-Being, 3*, 207–227.
Cropley, M., Ayers, S., & Nokes, L. (2003). People don't exercise because they can't think of reasons to exercise: An examination of causal reasoning within the Transtheoretical Model. *Psychology, Health & Medicine, 8*, 409–414.
Csikszentmihalyi, M. (1975/2000). *Beyond boredom and anxiety*. San Francisco: Jossey-Bass.
Csikszentmihalyi, M., & Massimini, F. (1985). On the psychological selection of bio-cultural information. *New Ideas in Psychology, 3*, 115–138.
Dash, V. B., & Junius, A. (1983). *A handbook of Āyurveda*. New Delhi: Concept Publishing Company.
Deci, E. L., & Ryan, R. M. (2000). The "what" and "why" of goal pursuits: Human needs and the self-determination of behavior. *Psychological Inquiry, 11*, 227–268.
Delle Fave, A. (2007). Individual development and community empowerment: Suggestions from studies on optimal experience. In J. Haworth & G. Hart (Eds.), *Well-being: Individual, community, and societal perspectives* (pp. 41–56). London: Palgrave McMillan.
Delle Fave, A. (2009). Optimal experience and meaning: Which relationship? *Psychological Topics, Special Journal Issue on Positive Psychology, 18*, 285–302.
Delle Fave, A. (2010). Development through disability: The unfolding and sharing of psychological resources. In G. W. Burns (Ed.), *Happiness, healing and enhancement: Your casebook collection for applying positive psychology in therapy* (pp. 88–99). Hoboken: Wiley.
Delle Fave, A. (2013a). Eudaimonic and Hedonic components of happiness. In A. Michalos (Ed.), *The encyclopedia of quality of life research*. Dordrecht: Springer.
Delle Fave, A. (2013b). Harmony. In A. Michalos (Ed.), *The encyclopedia of quality of life research*. Dordrecht: Springer.
Delle Fave, A., & Massimini, F. (2004). Bringing subjectivity into focus: optimal experiences, life themes and person-centred rehabilitation. In P. A. Linley & S. Joseph (Eds.), *Positive psychology in practice* (pp. 581–597). London: Wiley.
Delle Fave, A., & Massimini, F. (2005). The relevance of subjective wellbeing to social policies: Optimal experience and tailored intervention. In F. Huppert, B. Keverne, & N. Baylis (Eds.), *The science of wellbeing* (pp. 379–404). Oxford: Oxford University Press.
Delle Fave, A., Brdar, I., Freire, T., Vella-Brodrick, D., & Wissing, M. P. (2011a). The Eudaimonic and hedonic components of happiness: Qualitative and quantitative findings. *Social Indicators Research, 100*, 185–207.
Delle Fave, A., Massimini, F., & Bassi, M. (2011b). *Psychological selection and optimal experience across cultures. Social empowerment through personal growth*. Dordrecht: Springer Science.
Diener, E. (2000). Subjective well-being. *American Psychologist, 55*, 34–43.
Diener, E., Emmons, R. A., Larsen, R. J., & Griffin, S. (1985). The satisfaction with life scale. *Journal of Personality Assessment, 49*, 71–75.
Engel, G. L. (1977). The need for a new medical model: A challenge for biomedicine. *Science, 196*, 129–136.
Fava, G., & Ruini, C. (2003). Development and characteristics of well-being enhancing psychotherapeutic strategy: Well-being therapy. *Journal of Behavioural Therapy and Experimental Psychiatry, 34*, 45–64.

Feuerstein, G. (1998). *The Yoga-Sutra of Patanjali. A new translation and commentary*. Rochester: Inner Traditions International.
Fisher, K., & Johnston, M. (1996). Experimental manipulation of perceived control and its effect on disability. *Psychology and Health, 11*, 657–669.
Folkman, S., & Greer, S. (2000). Promoting psychological well-being in the face of serious illness: When theory, research and practice inform each other. *Psycho-Oncology, 9*, 11–19.
Frawley, D. (2004). *Yoga and Āyurveda*. Delhi: Motilal Banarsidass Publishers.
Fredrickson, B. L. (2001). The role of positive emotions in positive psychology: The broaden-and-build theory of positive emotions. *American Psychologist, 56*, 218–226.
Galvin, L. R., & Godfrey, H. P. D. (2001). The impact of coping on emotional adjustment to spinal cord injury (SCI): Review of the literature and application of a stress appraisal and coping formulation. *Spinal Cord, 39*, 615–627.
Gollwitzer, P., & Oettingen, G. (1998). The emergence and implementation of health goals. *Psychology & Health, 13*, 687–715.
Gregor, K., Zvolensky, M., Leen-Feldner, E., Yartz, A., & Feldner, M. (2006). Perceived health, a test of incremental validity in relation to smoking outcome expectancies, motivation to smoke and desire to quit smoking. *Cognitive Behaviour Therapy, 35*, 28–42.
Hankey, A. (2010). Establishing the scientific validity of Tridoṣa. Part I: Doṣa s, Subdoṣa s and Doṣa Prakritis. *Ancient Science of Life, 29*, 6–18.
Hurley, C. C., & Shea, C. A. (1992). Self-efficacy: Strategy for enhancing diabetes self-care. *The Diabetes Educator, 18*, 146–150.
Jenkins, R., & Pargament, K. (1995). Religion and spirituality as resources for coping with cancer. *Journal of Psychosocial Oncology, 13*, 51–74.
Joseph, S., & Linley, A. (2006). Growth following adversity: Theoretical perspectives and implications for clinical practice. *Clinical Psychology Review, 26*, 1041–1053.
Juyal, R. C., Negi, S., Wakhode, P., Bhat, S., Bhat, B., & Thelma, B. K. (2012). Potential of ayurgenomics approach in complex trait research: Leads from a pilot study on rheumatoid arthritis. *PLoS One, 7*(9), e45752. doi:10.1371/journal.pone.0045752.
Kahneman, D., Diener, E., & e Schwarz, N. (Eds.). (1999). *Well-being: The foundations of hedonic psychology*. New York: Russell Sage.
Keyes, C. L. M. (1998). Social well-being. *Social Psychology Quarterly, 61*, 121–140.
Keyes, C. L. M. (2003). Complete mental health: An agenda for the 21st century. In C. L. M. Keyes & J. Haidt (Eds.), *Flourishing: Positive psychology and the life well-lived* (pp. 293–312). Washington, DC: American Psychological Association.
Keyes, C. L. M. (2005). Mental illness and/or mental health? Investigating axioms of the complete state model of health. *Journal of Consulting and Clinical Psychology, 73*, 539–548.
Keyes, C. L. M. (2007). Promoting and protecting mental health as flourishing: A complementary strategy for improving national mental health. *American Psychologist, 62*(2), 95–108.
Keyes, C. L. M., Wissing, M., Potgieter, J. P., Temane, M., Kruger, A., & van Rooy, S. (2008). Evaluation of the Mental Health Continuum–Short Form (MHC–SF) in Setswana-speaking South Africans. *Clinical Psychology & Psychotherapy, 15*, 181–192.
Kipling, W., Forgas, J., & Von Hippel, W. (Eds.). (2005). *The social outcast: Ostracism, social exclusion, rejection, and bullying*. New York: Psychology Press.
Kiran Kumar, S. K. (2003). An Indian conception of well-being. In J. Henry (Ed.), *Proceedings of European Positive Psychology Conference* (pp. 538–551). Leicester: British Psychological Society.
Kiran Kumar, S. K. (2004). Perspectives on well-being in the Indian tradition. *Journal of Indian Psychology, 22*(2), 5–8.
Kiran Kumar, S. K. (2006). The role of spirituality in attaining well-being: Approach of Sanātana Dharma. In A. Delle Fave (Ed.), *Dimensions of well-being* (pp. 538–551). Milano: Franco Angeli.
Kreuter, M. (2000). Spinal cord injury and partner relationships. *Spinal Cord, 38*, 2–6.
Kuijer, R. G., & deRidder, D. T. D. (2003). Discrepancy in illness-related goals and quality of life in chronically ill patients: The role of self-efficacy. *Psychology and Health, 18*, 313–330.
Kuppuswami, B. (1985). *Elements of ancient Indian psychology*. Delhi: Konark Publishers.

Larson, D. B., Koenig, H. G., Kaplan, B. H., Greenberg, R. S., Logue, E., & Taylor, H. A. (1989). The impact of religion on men's blood pressure. *Journal of Religion and Health, 28*, 265–278.
Lazarus, R. S. (2000). Toward better research on stress and coping. *American Psychologist, 55*, 665–673.
Levin, B., & Browner, C. (2005). The social production of health: Critical contributions from evolutionary, biological, and cultural anthropology. *Social Science & Medicine, 61*, 745–750.
Massimini, F., & Delle Fave, A. (2000). Individual development in a bio-cultural perspective. *The American Psychologist, 55*, 24–33.
McClain, C. S., Rosenfeld, B., & Breitbart, W. (2003). Effect of spiritual well-being on end-of-life despair in terminally-ill cancer patients. *Lancet, 361*, 1603–1607.
McCullough, M. E., Larson, D. B., Hoyt, W. T., Koenig, H. G., & Thoreson, C. E. (1999). *Religious involvement and mortality: A meta-analysis review*. 107th Convention of the American Psychological Association, Boston, MA.
Mead, N., & Bower, P. (2000). Patient-centredness: A conceptual framework and a review of the empirical literature. *Social Science and Medicine, 51*, 1087–1110.
Mead, N., Bower, P., & Hann, M. (2002). The impact of general practitioner's patient-centredness on patients' post-consultation satisfaction and enablement. *Social Science & Medicine, 55*, 283–299.
Merluzzi, T. V., & Sanchez, M. A. (1997). Assessment of self-efficacy and coping with cancer: Development and validation of the cancer behavior inventory. *Health Psychology, 16*, 163–170.
Mytko, J. J., & Knight, S. J. (1999). Body, mind and spirit: Towards the integration of religiosity and spirituality in cancer quality of life research. *Psycho-Oncology, 8*, 439–450.
Omran, R. (1971). The epidemiologic transition: A theory of the epidemiology of population change. *Millbank Memorial Fund Quarterly, 49*, 509–538.
Pande, N., & Naidu, R. K. (1992). Anāsakti and health: A study on non-attachment. *Psychology and Developing Societies, 4*, 89–104.
Park, C., & Folkman, S. (1997). The role of meaning in the context of stress and coping. *Review of General Psychology, 1*, 115–144.
Patwardhan, B., & Bodeker, G. (2008). Ayurvedic genomics: Establishing a genetic basis for mind-body typologies. *Journal of Alternative and Complementary Medicine, 14*, 571–576.
Pennebaker, J. W. (1997). *Opening up: The healing power of expressing emotions*. New York: Guilford Press.
Prasher, B., Negi, S., Aggarwal, S., Mandal, A. K., Sethi, T. P., Deshmukh, S. R., et al. (2008). Whole genome expression and biochemical correlates of extreme constitutional types defined in Āyurveda. *Journal of Translational Medicine, 6*, 48.
Prochaska, J., & DiClemente, C. (1984). *The transtheoretical approach: Crossing the traditional boundaries of change*. Homewood: J. Irwin.
Prochaska, J., Velicer, W., Rossi, J., Marcus, B., Rakowsky, W., Fiore, C., Harlow, L., Redding, C., Rosenbloom, D., et al. (1994). Stages of change and decisional balance for 12 problem behaviors. *Health Psychology, 13*, 39–46.
Quarantelli, E. L. (1985). An assessment of conflicting views on mental health. The consequences of traumatic events. In C. R. Figley (Ed.), *Trauma and its wake* (pp. 173–215). New York: Brunner/Mazel.
Rolland, J. S., & Walsh, F. (2005). Systemic training for healthcare professionals: The Chicago Center for Family Health Approach. *Family Process, 44*, 283–301.
Ryan, R. M., & Deci, E. L. (2001). On happiness and human potentials: A review of research on hedonic and eudaimonic well-being. *Annual Review of Psychology, 52*, 141–166.
Ryan, R. M., Huta, V., & Deci, E. L. (2008). Living well: A self-determination theory perspective on eudaimonia. *Journal of Happiness Studies, 9*, 139–170.
Ryff, C. (1989). Happiness is everything, or is it? Explorations on the meaning of psychological well-being. *Journal of Personality and Social Psychology, 57*, 1069–1081.
Ryff, C. D., & Singer, B. H. (2008). Know thyself and become what you are: A eudaimonic approach to psychological well-being. *Journal of Happiness Studies, 9*, 13–39.
Schlegel, R. J., Hicks, J. A., King, L. A., & Arndt, J. (2011). Feeling like you know who you are: Perceived true self-knowledge and meaning in life. *Personality and Social Psychology Bulletin*. doi:10.1177/0146167211400424.

Sen, A. (1992). *Inequality reexamined.* Oxford: Oxford University Press.
Sharma, R. K., & Baghwan Dash. (1998). *Ćaraka Saṃhitā* (English translation, 7 vol.). Varanasi: Chowkhamba Sanskrit Series.
Sheldon, K., Williams, G., & Joiner, T. (2003). *Self-determination theory in the clinic: Motivating physical and mental health.* New Haven: Yale University Press.
Sirgy, M. J., & Wu, J. (2009). The pleasant life, the engaged life, and the meaningful life: What about the balanced life? *Journal of Happiness Studies, 10*, 183–196.
Sodergren, S. C., & Hyland, M. E. (2000). What are the positive consequences of illness? *Psychology and Health, 15*, 85–97.
Spencer, L., Pagell, F., Hallion, M., & Adams, T. (2002). Applying the transtheoretical model to tobacco cessation and prevention: A review of the literature. *American Journal of Health Promotion, 17*, 7–71.
Srikantha Murthy, K. R. (Ed.). (2007). *Vaghbata Astanga Hṛdaya m.* Varanasi: Chowkhamba Krishnadas Academy.
Stanton, A. L., Danoff-Burg, S., Cameron, C. L., Bishop, M., Collins, C. A., Kirk, S. B., Sworowski, L. A., & Twillman, R. (2000). Emotionally expressive coping predicts psychological and physical adjustment to breast cancer. *Journal of Consulting and Clinical Psychology, 68*, 875–882.
Subramanya Sastri, V. V. (2009). *Tridoṣa theory.* Kottakkal: Arya Vaidya Sala.
Swami Chinmayananda. (1952). *Discourses on Kenopanishad.* Bombay: Central Chinmaya Mission Trust.
Swami Chinmayananda. (1954). *Prasna Upanishad.* Bombay: Central Chinmaya Mission Trust.
Swami Chinmayananda. (1975). *The Holy Geeta. A commentary.* Bombay: Central Chinmaya Mission Trust.
Swami Chinmayananda. (1992). *Discourses on Taittiriya Upanishad.* Bombay: Central Chinmaya Mission Trust.
Thirumulpadu, V. K. R. (2010). *Glimpses of wisdom.* Bangalore: I-AIM.
Veenhoven, R. (2002). Why social policy needs subjective indicators? *Social Indicators Research, 58*, 33–45.
World Health Organization. (2001). *International classification of functioning, disability and health.* Endorsed by the Fifty-Fourth World Health Assembly for International use on May 22, 2001. http://www.who.int/icidh
World Health Organization. (2002). *The world health report 2002. Reducing risks, promoting healthy life.* http://www.who.int/whr/2002/en/index.html
Wu, C. (2009). Enhancing quality of life by shifting importance perception among life domains. *Journal of Happiness Studies, 10*, 37–47.

Chapter 10
The Emergence of Health in Complex Adaptive Systems: A Common Ground for Āyurveda and Western Science

Antonio Morandi and Antonella Delle Fave

10.1 Introduction

Western medicine is undergoing deep conceptual changes, in the attempt to fill the steadily increasing gap between the theoretical underpinnings of the scientific method and the complexity of the observed reality. The compelling evidence of the variety of expressions and multifaceted interactions of the social and individual determinants of health challenges the current biomedical perspective, still centered on the analytical investigation of isolated structures, functions, and mechanisms.

A growing amount of studies are showing the potential of system biology, an approach grounded into the theories of chaos and complex systems that provides an integrated view of the amazing intricacy of life, opening new perspectives to our understanding of health and disease (Hood and Flores 2012; Mazzocchi 2012). However, this integrated view is still far from being applicable to the daily clinical practice, due to the lack of an overarching conceptual framework. Contemporary science is split between the evidence of indeterminism, acausality, and non-localization of the basic elements of nature brought forth by physics on the one side and the phenomenic reality of biological systems undergoing ceaseless changes in time under the pressure of internal and external causes on the other side. The connection between these two contradictory aspects of reality is the core of a lively debate that calls into play philosophical worldviews and religious beliefs besides experimental evidence (Kaufman 2008).

A. Morandi (✉)
School of Ayurvedic Medicine, Ayurvedic Point, Milano, Italy
e-mail: dr.morandi@ayurvedicpoint.it

A. Delle Fave
Department of Pathophysiology and Transplantation, University of Milano, Milan, Italy
e-mail: antonella.dellefave@unimi.it

A. Morandi and A.N. Narayanan Nambi (eds.), *An Integrated View of Health and Well-being*, Cross-Cultural Advancements in Positive Psychology 5, DOI 10.1007/978-94-007-6689-1_10,

The major problem in this debate is the difficulty to integrate such a variety of contrasting evidences within the Western cultural view of discontinuity between domains of knowledge. An integrated perspective that overcomes these difficulties is offered by Āyurveda, the ancient traditional medicine of India, grounded into the Eastern view of the substantial interconnectedness of all aspects of reality. Āyurveda shows amazingly modern features (Morandi et al. 2010, and Chap. 1 of this volume), and its conceptual underpinnings can be fruitfully interpreted and explained to a skeptical Western audience through the theoretical framework of complex systems (Rioux 2012). Āyurveda is centered on an inclusive and dynamic conceptualization of health, considered as an emergent phenomenon arising from the interplay of different life components, at the physical, psychological, social, and spiritual levels. This conceptualization is strikingly close to WHO's definition of health as "a state of complete physical, mental and social well-being, and not merely the absence of disease or infirmity" (WHO 1978).

In this chapter, we will attempt to highlight the similarities between the Western conceptualization of nature and living systems and the Ayurvedic one. Needless to say, Āyurveda is a system of knowledge that was developed independently and much earlier than modern science. Therefore, our aim is to not reduce Āyurveda to a science in Western terms. We will rather attempt to highlight commonalities and differences between the two approaches. A clear distinction between these two perspectives must be maintained indeed, in order to escape the ethnocentric temptation to forcefully include any aspect of human knowledge into the Western interpretation framework. As concerns Āyurveda, this means to tribute respect and recognition to its philosophical and conceptual core, which in fact represents one of its distinctive and most salient features, allowing for the interpretation of any phenomenon within the realm of life from an unequivocally integrated perspective.

To this purpose, we will first briefly refer to the definition of health and disease in the Western and Ayurvedic views, highlighting their different conceptual underpinnings, and then we will show how similarities between the two approaches can be detected adopting a complex systems' perspective.

10.2 Health and the Western Worldview

Modern medicine is currently dominated by the biomedical model, which is strictly analytical and problem centered (Delle Fave and Massimini 2005; Chaps. 1 and 2 of this volume). Physicians pay attention to the specific symptoms reported by their patients, trying to ascribe them to a well-defined pathology related to a specific body organ or apparatus. A treatment for each specific disorder is thus envisaged, disregarding how patients' whole-body functioning, natural environment, social context, and subjective experience can influence the onset and the outcomes of disease. The limitations of this model were firstly pointed out by Engel (1977), a psychiatrist who formalized the bio-psycho-social model, focused on the patient as a person with a subjective interpretation of health, disease, and quality of life; as a carrier of a specific cultural background; and as a member of a particular society, that is, as a complex living system (a more articulated discussion of this topic is provided in Chaps. 1 and 9).

Engel's model actually echoes a core statement of the Declaration of Human Rights (1948), according to which health is a state of physical, psychological, social, and spiritual well-being, as well as the WHO's definition of health reported above. This definition, currently accepted by researchers, professionals, and institutions worldwide, indeed provides a laudably bio-psycho-social view of health as a complex phenomenon. At the same time, it shows a crucial weakness: it is not of practical use (Saracci 1997). Can any common person's health conditions satisfy the assumption of completeness? The WHO definition is to be appreciated for its utopian hope of the best imaginable life for every human being, but it does not correspond to the experience of any real person (Delle Fave and Fava 2011).

Moreover, WHO's definition of health is absolute. Health is either complete or it cannot be defined as health. The typical Western tendency toward polarization is clearly evident here. Objects, phenomena, and events investigated in any domain are usually classified and measured on ranges or continua built between two opposite poles, such as positive/negative, true/false, dynamic/static, global/local, and divisible/indivisible.

This aspect is particularly problematic if we consider that WHO's definition of health focuses on three different levels at which complete well-being should be identified – the physical, the psychological, and the social one. However, these levels are interconnected, and the evaluation of health may vary within the same individual across life stages, across individuals, across social conditions, and across cultures.

At the individual level, each person develops a subjective evaluation of well-being and health according to criteria such as values, beliefs, goal hierarchy, personality, and idiosyncratic style of interaction with the environmental opportunities (Delle Fave 2006). Physical health conditions only partially influence this evaluation. For example, Albrecht and Devlieger (1999) found that 54.3 % of people with serious disablement rated their quality of life as excellent or good. People currently sick or recovering from disease can easily identify positive consequences of their illness, such as improved interpersonal relationships, positive personality changes, and reappraisal and restructuring of life (Sodergren and Hyland 2000). Two persons with the same degree of physical health can have different levels of functioning and well-being. This depends upon variables unrelated to physical conditions but nevertheless connected with health: individual psychological features, family and social support, material and economic resources, educational background, cultural representations, and social policies (Ingstad 1999; Simeonsson et al. 2000; Űstün et al. 2001). At the social and cultural levels, research has widely demonstrated that persons with diseases or disabilities will only be disadvantaged in a social, cultural, or attitudinal environment in which their condition brings about disadvantageous consequences (Bickenbach et al. 1999).

Intrapersonal, interpersonal, and environmental factors therefore interact in moderating the effects of illness. A pivotal role is played by the opportunities for action and self-expression offered within the family life (Ünalan et al. 2001). In addition social relationships, education and job opportunities, architectonic and interpersonal facilitators, and barriers remarkably affect the quality of life of people with chronic or disabling pathologies (Meyers et al. 2002).

The impact of cultural trends and beliefs on health and related behaviors is particularly evident in postmodern societies. Improved living standards have brought forth longer life expectancy. Technological and scientific advancements allow people to survive and to attain a good quality of life in conditions that only few decades ago entailed death or dramatic constraints. In this context, patients expect to be offered solutions for any kind of problems, possibly by means of quick, time-saving remedies. Paradoxically, at the same time people of all ages engage in unhealthy but emotionally rewarding behaviors, such as substance abuse, excessive food intake or too severe diet restrictions, exposure to health risks in sports and sexual behaviors, and too much or too little physical exercise. For the abovementioned reasons, the growing investment on health in Western countries and – though less incisively – all over the world gave rise to an "epidemiological paradox." The increase in life expectancy led to an increase in the number of years spent living with chronic physical diseases and mental disorders, rather than greater health (Keyes 2007 and Chap. 1 of this volume).

This problem has been very acutely addressed by Sri Thirumulpadu, one of the most authoritative contemporary scholars in Āyurveda. He wrote "The current medical system is disease-centric … More medicines, more doctors, more hospitals only ensure more diseases … Despite increased morbidity, efficient emergency management has mitigated mortality. And morbidity reigns because of a bad philosophy of disease management which does not insist on a correct lifestyle" (2010, p. 51). The reason for this phenomenon, according to this scholar, lies in the lack of a philosophical system guiding the development of science.

10.3 Philosophy, Science, and Health: The Indian Perspective

The Indian culture developed a systematic and astonishingly deep knowledge about well-being and health, integrating the investigation of physiological processes and psychological functioning into the holistic perspective of the medical system of Āyurveda. However, in the Indian tradition the investigation of physiological and psychological functions and structures does not represent an independent knowledge domain. On the contrary, it is substantially related to philosophy and spirituality (Kuppuswami 1977; Rao 2008). According to Sri Thirumulpadu (2010) such a relationship is grounded into the role attributed to philosophy and science in the Indian tradition. *Darśana* or philosophy is generalized knowledge, offering a global view of life and concerned with differentiating between good and bad, well and ill. *Śāstra* or science is instead particularized knowledge, thus pertaining to practices and applications developed to ensure beneficial outcomes. The definition of health as a general and unitary human condition belongs to the domain of philosophy, while science has the specific role to find efficacious remedies to treat the particular and manifold conditions of disease.

Consistently with this view, the classical texts conveying the vision of Āyurveda – *Ćaraka Saṃhitā*, *Suśruta Saṃhitā*, and *Aṣṭāṇga Hṛdaya* – prominently follow the conceptualization of the *Sāmkhya* system. In particular the conceptualization and systematization of health and disease first developed by *Ćaraka* emerged from the complex interplay between different philosophical approaches, during a period of great intellectual ferment. The *Astika* or orthodox philosophical systems – *Mīmaṃsā*, *Upanishad* and *Advaita Vedānta*, *Sāmkhya*, *Yogā*, *Nyāya*, and *Vaiśeṣika* – based on the Vedic assumption of a universal and eternal consciousness principle were challenged by new *Nāstika*, or heterodox, systems – *Jainism* and *Buddhism* – that did not recognize Vedic authority and thus denied the existence of a consciousness principle (Swami Prabhavananda 1977). In the effort to provide a unified conceptualization of life, health, and disease, *Ćaraka* drew inspiration and information from both the *Astika* and *Nāstika* systems. Far from just borrowing ideas and concepts, however, he developed an original and articulated system of knowledge joining philosophy and science. "Philosophical winds blew through his mind but never lifted him off his feet from the bedrock of service to fellow beings" (Valiathan 2009, p. ii). The subsequent contributions of *Suśruta* and *Vagbhata* added elaboration and expansion to *Ćaraka's* system, without however modifying its core assumptions, solidly rooted into Indian philosophy.

According to the *Sāmkhya* conceptualization (also referred to in Chap. 3), followed since *Ćaraka* by most Āyurveda scholars, the universe stemmed from the interaction between the two eternal and unmanifest principles of *Puruṣa* – the consciousness principle, passive and unchangeable, and *Prakṛti* – the material principle, active and dynamic. This interaction led to the manifestation and differentiation of all living entities. Both unmanifest principles – eternal consciousness and material nature – are therefore embodied in each living being. *Ćaraka* provides a synthetic description of this evolution process from consciousness to manifestation. For example, in *Sūtra Sthāna* he states:

> There was never non-existence of the flow of life or intellect (Ćaraka Saṃhitā Sūtra Sthāna 30, 27 in Sharma and Dash 2001).

This conceptualization implies – among other aspects – the ontological identity between the individual soul (*Ātman*) and the universal consciousness principle (*Brahman*), both eternal and unchangeable:

> The embryo is produced of *ātman* (the self) ....known as jiva, eternal, not afflicted by diseases, old age, death and decay; not subjected to incision, excision, agitation, having universal forms and actions, unmanifest, beginning-less as well as endless and without any transformation. He entering into the uterus and combining with sperm and ovum produces himself in the form of embryo that is why the embryo is called as "the self." The birth of that self is not possible because of his beginning-lessness ... In fact, birth is only transformation in respect of age and conditions ... In spite of sperm, ovum, and the self, they do not attain the state of embryo until they are combined together; this comes into existence by combination. (Ćaraka Saṃhitā ŚārīraSthāna 3, 8 in Sharma and Dash 2001).

Consistently with this perspective, *Ćaraka* defines life – *Ayus*:

> Mind, self and body, these three make a tripod on which the living world stands. The (living body) is *Puruṣa* sentient and location of this *Veda* (Āyurveda). For him alone, this Veda is brought to light (Ćaraka Saṃhitā Sūtra Sthāna 1, 46–47 in Sharma and Dash 2001).

This description of life and of the individual is crucially different from the modern Western scientific approach that systematically separates biomedical knowledge (concerning the body) from psychology (concerning the mind) and theology or philosophy (concerning the soul). This substantial separation is common practice in spite of the bio-psycho-social model and the WHO's definition of health.

The interplay among the various levels of human functioning in promoting or hindering health is especially evident in the attention that Āyurveda scholars pay to the importance of a balanced attitude towards the fulfillment of individual needs and aspirations. Behavioral and psychological balance as the basic prerequisite for health and well-being is repeatedly emphasized by all the major Āyurveda scholars:

> The sense organs should neither be troubled very much nor should they be coaxed very much.

and

> In all dealings, one should adopt the middle mean only (Aṣṭāṇga Hṛdaya Sūtra Sthāna 2, 29–30 in Srikantha Murthy 2007a).

An effective synthesis of this interpretation of health can be found in *Suśruta Saṃhitā*. The term for health used here is *Svastha* that means "to be established (*Stha*) in oneself (*Sva*)":

> One whose physiological functions (*doṣa*), metabolism (agni), body tissues (*dhātu*) and excretory functions (*mala*) are in a state of equilibrium with cheerful mind, clarity of intellect and contented senses is said to be established in oneself (*swastha*) (Suśruta Saṃhitā Sūtra Sthāna 1, 15 in Srikantha Murthy 2007b).

Prasannata denotes happiness and equipoise. Health or *swasthya* is therefore defined as the equilibrium between anatomical, biological, physiological, mental, and spiritual components of the human being, involving the physical body (*sthula śārira*), the subtle body (*suksma śārira*), and the causal body (*karana śārira*), as described in detail in Chaps. 4 and 5 of this volume.

10.4 Life in the Western Perspective: Complexity, Chaos, and Coherence

Aristotle claimed that the whole is more than the sum of its parts. This is one of the founding concepts of the Western investigation of nature. The term complexity, first used by European scientists and philosophers in the eighteenth century, synthesizes the essence of this claim. It derives from the Latin verb complecti – "to encircle, embrace" – composed by the preposition com- "with" and the verb plectere "to weave, braid, twine." Living organisms are complex systems in that they are composed by different parts, each of them contributing to the system's functioning and adaptive interaction with the environment, by virtue of their integration as well as a specific differentiation in role and structure. Complexity is grounded into two peculiar features that characterize living systems: a far-from-equilibrium energetic structure, also labeled as negentropic (Ayers 1997; Duke 1994; Prigogine and Stengers 1984), and autopoiesis, or the intrinsic potential for self-organization (Maturana and Varela 1986). The process of development consists in an increase of the system's complexity, by virtue of the ceaseless exchange of information with the environment, thus introducing the concept of complex adaptive system (CAS) (Holland 1995, 1997, 1998; Couture 2007).

A CAS is therefore an integrated collection of components that dynamically and adaptively interact among each other and with the environment. The higher the system adaptability, the higher is its resilience in the presence of perturbations. Moreover, compared with inanimate physical entities, living systems are highly differentiated. Their components are specialized at the anatomical and physiological levels, each contributing to specific functions and being reciprocally connected in a coordinated pattern that allows for the adaptive interaction of the system with the environment (Tononi and Edelman 1998).

Miller (1970) summarized the features of complex negentropic systems by highlighting their statistical improbability: these systems are not derived from a casual interplay of elements but from a developmental process at least partly determined by the information embedded in the DNA. At the same time, living systems are predictable, thanks to their teleonomy (Monod 1971), defined as the intrinsic project that shapes their structures, functions, and stable features, as well as their behavioral alternatives in the interaction with the environment. Complex living systems have also been labeled as dissipative structures, in that the preservation and increase of their complexity require a ceaseless consumption of energy, partly transformed into activities and ordered structures and partly dissipated due to collateral phenomena (Nicolis and Prigogine 1989). Without a steady supply of energy, any complex system tends towards states of homogeneity, loss of specialization, disruption, and entropy. In living systems these states can be assimilated to decay and death.

The pattern of stable features of a system that can be observed, and that allows to identify the system as a well-defined entity, can be also interpreted as the coherence of the system itself. Coherence is a state in which the system can be observed as a whole integrated configuration, apparently "independent" of the environment. The highest state of coherence is characterized by minimal uncertainty, and it contributes to the predictability of living systems and their behavior (Couture 2007). However, due to the ceaseless interactions with the environment, the intrinsic developmental trends, and the varying amount of energy available to the system for its own maintenance and transformation, the level and expression of coherence undergoes changes, allowing for diverse system configurations.

A further peculiar feature of living systems, related to their adaptability and flexibility, is their potential for manifesting emergent properties, in other terms for creativity and innovation (Goldstein 1999; Fromm 2004, 2005). In the interaction process with the environment and its demands, a living system can develop adaptive behavioral strategies that were not previously part of its repertoire, or it can undergo structural modifications that make it better fit the environmental pressures. These processes and events allow for situating complex living systems beyond the realm of determinism and for conceptualizing emergence – of new properties, structures, and functions – as a distinctive aspect of the living world. In phylogeny, emergent properties are the core elements of speciation and, more generally, of biological evolution (Wilson 1975).

The above-described peculiarities of complex systems led to the development of a new mathematical approach that could adequately represent their functioning and dynamic adaptation tendency. This approach is grounded into Chaos Theory, a mathematical framework that overcomes the boundaries of the methods traditionally used to describe deterministic phenomena (Baranger 1999). Within this framework, living organisms are considered chaotic systems. They are characterized by nonlinearity, which implies a nonproportional relationship between input received and output produced. Chaotic systems are also highly sensitive to initial conditions, in that any minimal variation or perturbation, either internal or derived from their interaction with the environment, will multiply and spread its effects snowball-like, leading to unpredictable outcomes – such as emergent properties or behaviors.

When transposed into geometry, solutions of mathematic nonlinear equations result in fractals. Fractals are geometrical objects, characterized by a recursive and self-generating structure, as well as by intrinsic order and beauty. They can be used to describe the structure of leaves, nerve networks, or the circulatory system (Baranger 1999). Chaotic behavior has been detected in biological functions such as heart rhythm and brain waves, whose shape cannot be described through traditional geometrical models, due to their essential nonlinearity (Goldbergerer et al. 2002a). In nature chaotic systems are massively present. Actually, nature as a whole appears intrinsically chaotic.

In particular, any complex system is characterized by the presence of so-called chaotic or strange attractors. From a mathematical point of view, an attractor is defined as an infinite set of points to which orbits, trajectories, and events emanating from starting conditions tend in the course of the dynamic evolution of the system examined (Couture 2007). In a chaotic system, these trajectories are "strange," in that they are neither linear nor periodic. They rather tend to be unique, never repeating and never passing by the same point, though asymptotically close to each other. The graphic representation of strange attractors shows bifurcations and convolutions, folding and unfolding patterns that undergo changes consistent with the system evolution and adaptation. Strange attractors can be considered specific patterns of internal organization of the system, characterized by intrinsic sets of rules and properties that can shape structures and functions of smaller or larger portions of the system itself. The pervasive sharing of the same set of rules and properties across the various parts of a system corresponds to a high level of coherence of the system.

Finally, a living being is not an isolated entity, occasionally interacting with the environment. It is rather part of it, as an essential component of the net of relationships that constitutes the environment itself and that undergoes changes and transformation. From this perspective, nature is an articulated web of complex systems in dynamic interaction and transformation. These ceaseless interactions imply that each component of the systems at any level of observation (cells in an organ, organs in a body, organisms in an environment) undergoes continuous changes, fluctuating between negentropic and entropic tendencies and dynamically pursuing the highest possible levels of stability and coherence. The modern Western attempt to study nature by isolating its components has fostered the development of distinct domains of knowledge – physics, biology, chemistry, psychology – each of them investigating single aspects of an articulated web of complex systems. Researchers have acquired a vast amount of information about these specific aspects – the elementary structure, the molecular one, and the function of single organs or apparatuses – to the detriment of an integrated view. All these specific aspects are in fact embedded into the organisms' complex functioning and organization, from which their configuration itself derives. Body organs do not exist as such: the body is one and every piece is part of it, and it is determined in structure and function by the whole system's teleonomy and adaptation trend.

Moreover, additional complex systems emerged from the biological ones. Culture emerged from natural selection on the basis of peculiar biological features of the human species, developing with time into a complex system itself, characterized by intrinsic rules and patterns, and interacting with biology in the shaping of human behavior (Boyd and Richerson 1985; Delle Fave et al. 2011; Jablonka and Lamb 2005). Conscious experience emerges from the moment-by-moment integration of functional clusters of neurons – labeled dynamic cores – that selectively interact (Tononi and Edelman 1998). Each specific state of consciousness arising from this interaction represents one possibility among billions of others, showing a chaotic pattern characterized by a peculiar configuration of neural activities that reduces uncertainty and therefore can be considered an ordered and negentropic entity. Moreover, "experience may arise from the physical, but it is not entailed by the physical" (Chalmers 1995, p. 208), thus implying the emergent nature of the psychological realm. Complexity and related concepts have proved to be heuristically relevant also in the analysis of human communities and social organizations (Eldredge and Grene 1992; Khalil and Boulding 1996).

These evidences provide a view of reality as a web of complex systems developing and interacting at multiple levels. The paradigm shift necessary to understand it requires not only to consider all the interconnections among the components of each single system but also all the levels of complexity and the dynamic relationships characterizing the environment with which the specific system interacts.

10.5 Āyurveda and Complexity

The representation of reality that characterizes Āyurveda well fits the theories of chaos, complexity, and complex systems.

As reported in the previous section, according to *Sāmkhya* the whole universe emerges from the primordial interaction between the eternal and unmanifest principles of *Puruṣa* and *Prakṛti*. *Prakṛti* is the eternal principium of existence, the background of all manifestations. It can be described as a balanced mixture of the three basic qualities that characterize the perceivable world, called *Maha Guṇa* (great qualities): *Sattva* – balance and intelligence; *Rajas* – acceleration, dynamic and transformational energy; and *Tamas* – deceleration, inertia. According to *Sāmkhya* these qualities are in fact the substantive entities that compose any manifestation of reality, be it mental or physical. *Prakṛti* however is totally devoid of characteristics and thus indeterminate, indefinite, and lacking of coherence (Dasgupta 1924). This is due to the fact that in *Prakṛti* the *Guṇa* are reciprocally neutralized in a balanced and "homogeneous" pattern, so that none of them is manifest. This condition of global balance represents a seminal state of infinite potentiality, open to developing into any possible manifestation, containing the seed of all possible configurations of the perceivable reality (Guénon 1932).

It is worthy noticing that the *Sāmkhya* view considers *Prakṛti* not as a simple substance but as the totality of *guṇa* in their state of reciprocal counter-opposition. Apart from *Guṇa* there is no *Prakṛti*. *Prakṛti* as the equilibrium of the three *Guṇa* is the absolute ground of all the mental and phenomenal modifications – pure potentiality in which no complex qualities are manifested. In fact, this condition of equilibrium is not a mere passive state, but one of utmost tension; there is intense activity, but the activity here does not lead to the generation of new things and qualities (Dasgupta 1922).

It is also important to clarify that in this view *Guṇa* are substances and not mere qualities. In the *Sāmkhya* qualities do not exist by themselves; each unit of quality is but a unit of substance without mass. In other words quality is but a particular manifestation or appearance of a subtle entity. Things do not possess quality, but quality signifies merely the pattern in which a substance behaves and reacts. Perceivable objects apparently possess many qualities, but "corresponding to each and every new unit of quality, however fine and subtle it may be, there is a corresponding subtle entity, the reaction of which is interpreted by us as a quality" (Dasgupta 1922, vol.1, p. 261).

The interaction of *Prakṛti* with *Puruṣa* – the eternal and unmanifest consciousness principle – gives rise to the manifestation of the cosmos, that fulfills the purpose of the *Puruṣa* to fully enjoy experiences and to be released and liberated from them. This introduces a conscious orientation into the intrinsic but nondirectional tension of *Prakṛti*, breaking the balance between opposite *Guṇa* and leading to systems characterized by progressively increasing levels of organization, differentiation, and complexity.

In this process of transformation, the three *Guṇa* interact in a variety of different patterns and configurations, thus evolving from the indefinite and qualitatively indeterminate condition of *Prakṛti* to progressively more definite and qualitatively determinate states. As clearly explained by Dasgupta (1922), though cooperating to produce the manifest world, they never coalesce. A particular *Guṇa* can become predominantly manifest in a specific phenomenon, while the others become latent. In particular, the feature of energy in the manifest reality is due to the element of Rajas; the features of resistance and stability are due to Tamas; all conscious manifestation derives from Sattva.

The first system evolving from the *Puruṣa-Prakṛti* interaction and subsequent imbalance in the *Guṇa* interplay is characterized by a prominence of the *Sattva Guṇa*. As clarified by Dasgupta (1922), this system possesses the widest and most universal existence and is thus called *Mahat* (the great one), the universal order or intelligence. Subsequent modifications in the pattern of interaction among the *Guṇa* within *Mahat* give rise to the individual *Ahamkara*, characterized by the predominance of one *Guṇa* over the other two, thus contributing to shape the determinate structure of individual typologies. In fact the term *Ahamkara* means "what keeps building the image of self," that emphasizes the dynamic and transformational nature of this system. A ceaseless process of change indeed characterizes the individual's self-perception, based on the moment-by-moment fluctuation of the different *Maha Guṇa* and of their combination across a variety of patterns, depending on internal as well as environmental pressures.

In the further evolution steps, a twofold process is envisaged: on the one hand, the combination of *Sattva* and *Rajas* produces 11 different patterns of organization, classified as subtle substances and instrumental to the interaction with the material realm: five sense instruments (*Jnanendriya*), five action instruments (*Karmendriya*), and *Manas*, the mind, with the role of coordinating the *Indriya's* activities.

On the other hand, the interaction between *Tamas* and *Rajas*, between dynamism and staticity, and between acceleration and deceleration gives rise to five *Tanmātrā*, primordial units of matter that can be perceived by the *Indriya*.

> Matter is the place where *Guṇa* (qualities) and *Karma* (action) are inherent (Ćaraka Samitha Sūtra Sthāna 1, 50–51 in Sharma and Dash 2001)

The relation between *Rajas* and *Tamas* is well exposed as cause of recombination and separation which is the definition of *Karma* (action) as per *Ćaraka Samitha, Sūtra Sthāna* 1, 52 (in Sharma and Dash 2001).

The predominance of the *Tamas*, substantial inertia, allows for the manifestation of perceptible mass; the interaction of *Tamas* with *Rajas*, substantial dynamicity, leads to the manifestation of matter units, characterized by both mass and activity, the core features of any living system in the realm of biology.

The emergence of *Tanmātrā* represents the transition from the domain of unmanifest reals to the domain of manifest elements. The word *Tanmātrā* literally means "what is measurable," evoking the smallest particle of detectable matter. At this level, the first manifested entity is *Shabda*, the sound, bearing the primordial information of matter, namely, space occupancy and spatial relationship resulting in movement. *Shabda* is sequentially followed by four progressively more qualified and determined *Tanmātrā*, each of them encompassing the features of the previous *Tanmātrā*, as well as its own peculiarities: *Sparsha*, the touch, or potentiality of contact; *Rupa*, the shape, or potentiality of structure; *Rasa*, the taste, or potentiality of pervasion; and finally *Gandha*, the smell, or potentiality of subtle relationships.

The preponderance of *Tamas* within *Tanmātrā* finally gives rise to the *Mahābhūta*, or great elements: *ākash* (ether), *vāyu* (air), *tejas* (fire), *ap* (water), and *pṛthvi* (earth), five states of matter that, like *Tanmātrā*, derive one from the other in an evolutionary cascade and constitute the entire material realm.

To summarize, the *Mahābhūta* are manifest material states comprising the potentialities of *Tanmātrā* that in turn represent manifestations of *Maha Guṇa*. The structure and functions of each *Mahābhūta* are related to its material density level, from the lowest level in *Ākash* to the highest one in *pṛthvi*, in which *Tamas* is prominently manifest. This relationship highlights the inextricable intermingling of structure and function that occurs in any living system. Interestingly, the word *Mahābhūta* is composed by *Maha* (great) and *bhūta*, meaning "that which is," "true," but also "demon," "spirit." The substantial link between function and structure, quality and quantity, and energy and matter is embedded in this term.

10.5.1 Guruvadi Guṇa

As stated above, according to *Sāmkhya, Guṇa* are substances and not merely features of substances. Moving from the unmanifest level of *Maha Guṇa* to the manifest level of material entities, new *Guṇa* arise, progressively more determined and more physical in their manifestation.

In order to provide a description of living systems that could be useful and functional to the practical treatment purposes of Āyurveda, the ancient scholars and first of all *Ćaraka* paid prominent attention to the 20 *Guruvadi Guṇa* (literally "qualities related to heavy matter"), 10 couples of opposite physical qualities constitutive of any living system: cold-hot, dry-unctuous, heavy-light, gross-subtle, static-dynamic, dense-loose, rough-smooth, hard-soft, dull-penetrating, and viscous-fluid. *Guruvadi Guṇa* primarily and exhaustively represent the perceivable aspects of the variety of patterns of material aggregations, the *Pañca Mahābhūta*. As constituents of the manifest realm, *Guruvadi Guṇa* derive from specific patterns of combination between *Rajas* and *Tamas*; they provide information on the structure, functions, and reactions of the organism they belong to. Interestingly, one of the Sanskrit meaning of *Guṇa* besides "quality" is "rope," suggesting the role of *Guṇa* as links between the eternal and unmanifest consciousness and the material world.

Adopting a complex systems' perspective, the set of *Guruvadi Guṇa* that characterizes a living organism can be understood as expression of a far-from-equilibrium negentropic pattern of organization. This set of qualities or properties undergoes changes based on both the initial conditions of their manifestation and the ceaseless interaction of the living system with the environment and its pressures. The higher the internal coherence of the system, in terms of stability of relationships and interaction patterns among *Guṇa*, the more defined and determinate is the identity of the system as perceived by external observers.

10.5.2 Doṣa

As repeatedly highlighted, in the traditional Indian worldview, the manifest reality emerges from basic qualitative units and their reciprocal interactions. Consistently with this view, Āyurveda describes the human being – as the prominent target of its intervention – as a complex manifestation of *Guṇa's* interplay and transformation. The focus of Āyurveda is thus not the organism as a set of specific and materially observable parts or organs, but the variety of manifestation patterns of the *Guṇa*, as perceivable in the structure, functions, and behaviors of the individual.

Since *Guṇa* do not manifest themselves in isolation but through their reciprocal interactions and their effects on the organism's material structure and functioning, Āyurveda scholars developed a heuristically very powerful concept: the *Doṣa*. *Doṣa* are coherent and integrated ensembles of *Guruvadi Guṇa*, expressing general functional patterns of the organism as well as the related *Mahābhūta*, or matter constituents. Three *Doṣa* are identified in Āyurveda: *Vata Doṣa*, expression of the interplay between *ākash* (ether) and *vāyu* (air), and of their constitutive *Guruvadi Guṇa*; *Pitta Doṣa*, expression of the interaction between *tejas* (fire) and *ap* (water), and of the related *Guṇa*; and *Kapha Doṣa*, expression of the interplay between *ap* (water) and *pṛthvi* (earth), and of their *Guṇa*.

Considering that *Guṇa* are not stable entities but undergo ceaseless changes, *Doṣa* are dynamic systems in permanent transformation as well. The word *Doṣa* actually means "what is easily alterable; defect, perturbation," pointing to the instability of these systems. *Ćaraka* calls them as "pathogenic factors of the body" (Ćaraka Samitha Sūtra Sthāna I, 57 in Sharma and Dash 2001). At the same time, *Doṣa* represent coherent groupings of *Guruvadi Guṇa* and *Mahābhūta*, showing well-defined and typical features and thus allowing for their description as determined functional entities.

In each *Doṣa* the proportions of *Guruvadi Guṇa* and *Mahābhūta* are not fixed and stable, leading to a wide range of property manifestations. Nevertheless, since each *Doṣa* is expression of the interplay among specific *Guṇa* and *Mahābhūta*, its features and manifestations are also determined and contribute to the definition of the functions and influence pattern of the specific *Doṣa* on the whole living system's structure and functioning. More specifically, *Vata Doṣa* represents movement in all its forms – from bowel motion to breath and cardiovascular dynamics – thanks to its features of coldness, dryness, lightness, roughness, fluidity, and subtlety at the *Guṇa* level and of *ākash* and *vāyu* at the *Mahābhūta* level. *Pitta Doṣa* presides metabolic and transformational processes by virtue of its features of heat, lightness, softness, and fluidity at the *Guṇa* level and of *tejas* and *ap* at the *Mahābhūta* level. Finally, *Kapha* is the manifestation of the system's stability and cohesion, based on its *Guṇa-related* properties of staticity, grossness, density, coldness, dullness, and heaviness and on its *Mahābhūta* constituents *pṛthvi* and *ap* (Ćaraka Saṃhitā Sūtra Sthāna 1, 57 in Sharma and Dash 2001).

The concept of strange attractor developed in the complex systems' theoretical framework is very helpful to clarify the role of the *Doṣa*. *Doṣa* emerge from the nonlinear chaotic behavior of the *Guṇa/Mahābhūta* system, each of them representing a well-defined and coherent functional pattern evolved within the system's adaptation process. As strange attractors with n-dimensions – where "n" is the number of their property expressions, or *Guruvadi Guṇa* – each *Doṣa* funnels fluctuations in specific domains of the system, as well as specific structural or functional behaviors into nonlinear patterns of organization, thus providing flexibility to the system's adaptation trend. Moreover, the concept of *Doṣa* as entities that easily get out of balance explicitly accounts for their sensitivity to both internal and external perturbations. In fact, from this perspective *Doṣa* themselves behave chaotically, since their manifestation and impact on the whole system's conditions depend on the organism conditions, within a feedback loop process whose ultimate meaning is the preservation of an optimal level of balance in the system, matched with an optimal level of adaptation to the environmental demands.

The analogy between *Doṣa* and chaotic attractors is supported by the evidence of their extreme sensitivity to initial condition (Eckman and Ruelle 1985; Holden and Muhamad 1986). A slight perturbation in the relationships between the constitutive elements of the organism produces a remarkable change in *Doṣa* manifestation. In Āyurveda the imbalance of *Doṣa* is the first stage of disease, deriving from a perturbation in the *Guṇa* conditions.

10.5.3 Dhātu, Agni, and Energy Sources

In Āyurveda *Dhātu* are considered as the structural bases of an organism. Although the term *Dhātu* is often translated as "tissue elements," it rather means "that which sustains the body" from the root *Daa* (dha) "support, that which bears," conveying a more functional and less morphological representation of *Dhātu*.

In the classical Āyurveda texts, seven *Dhātu* are described, derived from different combinations of *Guṇa* and sequentially evolving one from the other, through a progressive increase in complexity and morpho-functional specificity. The first *Dhātu* is *Rasa*, the watery and least complex component of the organism, qualitatively defined as pervading, nourishing, and cohering liquid. The term *Rasa* has numerous meanings, many of them referring to harmony and embracing and suggesting all-encompassing potentiality. The second is *Rakta*, translated as blood and referring only to its particulate component, but whose meaning include "color red," "passionate," and "attached," suggesting reaction, contact, and connection. The third is *Māṃsa*, translated as "meat" but also "worm" and "time," suggesting movement, flow, and change. The fourth and most important *Dhātu* is *Meda*, fat: lipids in fact represent the key structural component of cells, organs, and organisms as a whole. The fifth is *Asthi*, or bone, meaning also "standing," "to resist"; the sixth one is *Majja*, the bone marrow, but meaning also "sinking" and "diving" which accounts for the depth of the anatomical location but also for the functional depth being the bone marrow related to staminal cells. The seventh and most complex *Dhātu* is *Śukra*, meaning semen, but also "juice," "essence of anything," and "good action."

The dynamic interaction of *Dhātu* through an evolving pattern is mediated by the action of *Agni*, the power of digestion and transformation (Ćaraka Saṃhitā Cikitsasthana 15, 1–16 in Sharma and Dash 2001).

Agni is the Vedic two-headed god of fire, representing the link between heaven and earth, the messenger between gods and humans. In this connecting role, it emerges from *Pitta Doṣa*, whose contrasting properties of hotness and dryness, on the one side, and coolness and sliminess/unctuousness, on the other side, are related to its constitutive *Mahābhūta*, *Tejas*, and *Ap*, respectively. The interaction between these contrasting *Guṇa* results in the emerging feature of instability that characterizes *Agni*. In its turn, Agni induces instability in any configuration pattern it gets in touch with, leading it to transformation. In the case of *Dhātu*, Agni leads to the gradual emergence of more complex patterns of organization from less complex ones. In this milieu of stabilization/destabilization of the *Dhātu* coherence, ultimately based on the reassembling and change of their *Guṇa*, other minor coherent entities emerge: the *upadhātu*, functional and structural transitional forms of *Dhātu* showing extreme and rigid pattern of coherence that do not allow them to undergo any further transformation, and the *mala*, or waste products (Ćaraka Saṃhitā Cikitsasthana 15, 15–35 in Sharma and Dash 2001).

Dhātu show a peculiar behavior, in that they tend to revert to normalcy "irrespective of any external causative factor" (Dasgupta 1922). This suggests the existence of a range of fluctuation in the *Dhātu* organization around a stability point far from the thermodynamic equilibrium, thus implying a resilience pattern that is typical of complex adaptive systems (Couture 2007) and that allows them to absorb and/or neutralize external perturbations, successfully adapting to environmental changes. Resilience is primarily due to the self-organizing features of the system, in particular to the redundancy of inner interdependent pathways and relationships that enhance the system's flexibility and variety of adaptation strategies. Resilience can be also defined as the autonomous healing capability of an organism that retrieves its original state of health after a remarkable perturbation, such as an injury or an environmental modification.

If the specific situation prevents the system from achieving a complete recovery, a new state of balance will be nevertheless attained, characterized by organization patterns and coherence levels differing from those typical of the original healthy state. This is exactly what happens in complex adaptive systems, when perturbed beyond their ability to retrieve their original state. In modern medical terms, it corresponds to the condition of chronic disease or to the aging process. In both cases irreversible changes occur in the system's physiological and structural pattern of organization, giving rise to a new and more or less stable condition of balance.

Within the conceptual framework of complex systems, *Dhātu* could be explained as specific material configuration patterns manifesting specific *Guṇa* and functions. However, this definition and the definition of *Doṣa* substantially overlap. Where does the distinction between *Dhātu* and *Doṣa* lie? Suśruta himself stated that "when normally functioning, the *Doṣa* constitute the body and are called *Dhātu*; when out of balance they create disease and discomfort and they are called *Doṣa*" (Bishagratna 1907). In Suśruta *Saṃhitā* the healthy state of an individual is defined as *TriDhātu*, and *Dhātu* represents the stable version of *Doṣa* (Dasgupta 1922; Bishagratna 1907). The same description is provided in Rig Veda (*Rigveda Saṃhitā*, I, 3, 6 as cited in Bishagratna 1907). It could be argued that the difference between *Dhātu* and *Doṣa* lies in the emphasis on structure versus function: *Dhātu* are expressions of the system's structural patterns, while *Doṣa* are expressions of the system's functional patterns. Nevertheless, a clear demarcation between the two is not possible, since the constitutive elements of both *Doṣa* and *Dhātu* are ultimately the three *Maha Guṇa*. In fact, analogous to what happens for *Doṣa*, the balance of *Dhātu* is considered essential for the preservation of health. Ćaraka states, "The very object of Āyurveda is the maintenance of the equilibrium of the *Dhātu*" (Ćaraka Saṃhitā Sūtra Sthāna 1, 53 in Sharma and Dash 2001).

It is therefore reasonable to assume that *Dhātu* represent the optimal coherence state of the *Doṣa* in their role of strange attractors: highly coherent *Doṣa* attain a high level of stability within their dynamic and negentropic organization pattern. This situation is coincident with an optimal function of the whole organism. It ultimately entails coherence in the *Guruvadi Guṇa* setup, leading to a complex and ordered morpho-functional pattern called *Dhātu*, whose main property is the capability to "sustain" the whole systems preserving its stability and integrity. *Dhātu* are thus the structural and functional expression of the organism in its healthy state and optimal function. This is consistent with the *Ćaraka's* statement "Disease is disequilibrium of the *Dhātu*. Health is equilibrium of *Dhātu*. Health is known as pleasure. Disease is known as pain." (Ćaraka Saṃhitā Sūtra Sthāna 9, 4 in Sharma and Dash 2001).

The level of organization and coherence of the individual, considered as a complex living system derived from the nonlinear interplay of *Guṇa* giving rise to *Mahābhūta*, *Doṣa*, and *Dhātu*, is maintained through a ceaseless intake of energy. Energy is necessary to promote the system's far-from-equilibrium stability, the related dissipation, and the elimination of substances that threaten the system's negentropic organization. The energy intake generally occurs through food, while the potentially destabilizing elements to be eliminated are by-products of the internal transformation processes, called *Mala* in Āyurveda, whose organization pattern does not fit the system's coherence anymore. Due to the substantial interconnection among *Doṣa*, *Dhātu*, and *Mala*, these three aspects cooperate to define the overall health condition of the organism (Ćaraka Saṃhitā Sūtra Sthāna 28, 1–5 in Sharma and Dash 2001).

The system's autopoiesis and self-organization result in a coherent behavior shaped and oriented by *Guṇa* and *Doṣa*; the latter, in their role of strange attractors, are defined in their specific features by internal relationships, rules, and functional patterns. However, without a continuous energy supply, *Guṇa* cannot maintain their coherence that corresponds to *Dhātu*. In this condition the *Doṣa* configuration, characterized by perturbation rather than stability, becomes prevalent. Interestingly, one of the Sanskrit words used in *Āyurveda* to indicate the body – *śārira* – literally means "what keeps decaying" suggesting the continuous struggle between destruction and construction, and catabolism and anabolism.

The balance between food intake and waste elimination is also crucial for maintaining health. The key role in this interaction is played by *Agni*, the transformative and destabilizing factor that assures the conversion of heterologous items into homologous ones, ultimately leading to the stabilization of the main system, through the creation of new components and the expulsion of unnecessary ones (waste) (Ćaraka Saṃhitā Cikitsasthana XV, 16–20 in Sharma and Dash 2001).

Within this context, it is interesting to specify what is food in Āyurveda. The Sanskrit word for food – *ahāra* – also means "fetching," "bringing near," "taking," "livelihood," and "use," thus comprising nutrition as well as, more generally, the act of contact and interaction. *Ahāra* represents every heterologous item that can be transformed into a homologous one through *Agni*, thus including any environmental stimulus that "feeds" the sense organs. Within this view, food is the environment itself. The act of living is an act of nutrition. This is consistent with the importance that Āyurveda attributes to the individual's relationship with the environment as the primary action of prevention.

10.5.4 Ojas or Emerging Health

The state of optimal health, derived from the global coherence and balanced organization of *Dhātu*, is ultimately expressed through *Ojas*. Ayurvedic classical text describe *Ojas* as the essence of *Dhātu*, deriving from their correct and coherent functioning (Ćaraka Saṃhitā Sūtra Sthāna XVII, 73–74 in Sharma and Dash 2001). *Ojas* is a complex and multidimensional concept, and its translation in Western words and meanings is extremely difficult. *Ojas* derives from the Sanskrit root *vaj* "strong," and it can be translated as "vigor," "strength," "vitality," "luster," and "manifestation," terms suggesting a function emerging from a background. The concept of *Ojas* is a manifestation of overall health, a measure of *Dhātu* coherence and organization and the resilience capacity of an organism. Overall, it is the ultimate expression of the multilevel functioning of the whole organism as a complex adaptive system. *Ojas* at its optimal level is the manifestation of a system characterized by high levels of complexity, in terms of inner coherence, organization, and, above all, resilience. If, for some reason, complexity is compromised because of the disruption in the network of events and elements that determine the system coherence, the resilience level decreases as well. The lower the resilience level, the more difficult it will be to restore the original complexity of the system after perturbations. This will eventually lead to a shift of the system towards a stable state, however, characterized by lower levels of complexity and resilience and consequently more fragile.

In line with this interpretation, *Ojas* is also commonly associated with the immune system. The key role of immunity – protection of the organism from external aggressions – is in fact consistent with the definition of *Ojas* as the overall capability of the system to adapt and to be resilient, that arises from the balance and coherence among its components.

This view is consistent with what is commonly observed in chronic diseases and in the process of aging where, according to Āyurveda, the level and quality of *Ojas* become suboptimal. The loss of *Ojas* integrity, corresponding to a reduction in the organism's functional and structural complexity, will result in a lower adaptation potential. Low physiological complexity is an indicator of a relatively simple control system, showing low adaptability under perturbation, and thus higher vulnerability to the environmental stressors (Manor et al. 2010; Manor and Lipsitz 2012). Loss of complexity and simplification of physiological pathways represent typical features of many diseases as well as of the aging process (Goldbergerer et al. 2002b; Kyriazis 2003; Mangel 2001). Aging is associated with a progressively decreasing rate of dendrite formation in the brain (Schierwagen 1987), a lower complexity of EEG activity (Skinner et al. 1992), and a decline of heart rate variability (Kaplan et al. 1991; Kresh and Izrailtyan 1998). In diseases involving the motor system, such as Parkinson's, arthritis, and stroke, a progressive decrease of complexity is observed in the movement range (Edwards et al. 1999) and in gait dynamics (Hausdorff et al. 1997). In patients with Alzheimer's disease, the EEG pattern is slower and less complex that the pattern observed in age-matched healthy people (Dauwels et al. 2011). In diabetes mellitus type 2, there is a progressive loss of complexity in the glycemic profile, in association with other markers of disease progression (Churruca et al. 2008).

On the opposite pole of life, namely, fetus formation, *Ojas* is considered a crucial element as well, representing a measure of the positive outcome of the mother-child exchanges (including exchange of *Ojas* itself) taking place during pregnancy (Dasgupta 1922). *Ojas* is therefore the most general expression of the organism's coherence, organization, and complexity, largely overlapping the currently accepted conceptualization of health.

10.6 The Health Continuum

The word Āyurveda includes the term *Ayus*, which means both life and health. Āyurveda can thus be translated as knowledge/science of life and knowledge/science of health. The most comprehensive manifestation and measure of health is *Ojas* that corresponds to the capacity of an organism to survive in an optimal state successfully adapting to the environmental conditions and changes. Within this view, health represents a dynamic process rather than a discrete condition, ranging from optimal to poor. "Optimal health" as strong *Ojas* emerges from the coherence of *Guṇa* and *Dhātu* as the most global expression of the system's complexity. It reflects the system's ability to successfully adapt to the environmental demands through the ceaseless process of adjustment and coordination among structures and functions that allows the system to maintain an optimal balance or to retrieve it after intense solicitations. Conversely, "poor health" is a condition of inability to restore the system's original level of complexity after exposure to stressors. In the condition of poor health, or poor *Ojas*, the system can find a new relative stability at a lower level of complexity characterized by reduced *Ojas*, and thus reduced health, as what happens in chronic diseases or aging. The whole negentropic organization of the system is modified, with the definition of new patterns, limits, and resilience levels. Finally, the extreme condition of "absent health" corresponds to the complete disruption of the system's coherence and complexity, corresponding to the biological concept of death.

From this perspective, health is a continuously variable condition, rather than a well-defined and discrete one. It reaches the optimal level when all system's functions and structures cooperate coherently and effectively, through highly complex patterns of interactions. This balance gets however continuously disrupted by the interaction with the environment, thus requiring a ceaseless readjustment process of the whole system, whose effectiveness is represented by resilience. The wider is the range of modifications and pressures that the system can absorb, being able to subsequently retrieve optimal levels of health, the stronger is its resilience. However, when the intensity of pressures or stressors overcomes the resilience limits, the system starts manifesting functional alterations giving rise to a new state globally acknowledged as disease. In this situation, external interventions known as therapies are needed, in order to bring the system's functioning back to a more complex and resilient pattern of organization. Old age, fatigue, resource exhaustion, or other conditions characterized by lower *Ojas* and resilience induce stable states of suboptimal health – or disease – as reactions to stressors and pressures that are otherwise tolerated as sources of only temporary imbalance.

The main goal of Āyurveda as a medical system is to keep the individual system's resilience at the highest possible level, in order to guarantee adaptation and optimal health in the face of even very large fluctuations of environmental demands and stressors. This is the purpose of the preventive practices known as *Swasthavritta*. *Swastha* means healthy and *Vritta* means correct behavior, referring to the daily or seasonal hygienic routines and overall lifestyle that promote optimal health. The health status of each person depends therefore upon their awareness of life as a continuous process in which every action influences the general psychophysical balance and complexity.

From a broader perspective, individual health behaviors are connected through a relation of reciprocal causality with social values and customs (Delle Fave 2010), as described in Sect. 10.2. Healthy individuals build healthy communities, whereas unhealthy lifestyles can generate negative consequences in the balance of society as a complex system itself. In their turns, cultural norms and practices play a pivotal role in promoting citizens' healthy or unhealthy behaviors (Delle Fave and Massimini 2005; Morandi et al. 2011).

10.7 The Implications of Āyurveda for Health Promotion

The conceptualization of health in Āyurveda has several relevant implications at both the conceptual and practical levels.

First of all, health as a dynamic condition can achieve stable configurations at different levels of complexity, including states labeled as disease and death. In this view disease is not a discrete entity, opposed to health. The various factors that influence the level of health, and thus complexity of an organism, play a prominently regulatory role rather than being direct and univocal causes of health, on the one side, and disease, on the other side. According to their quantitative and qualitative features, as well as according to the conditions of the organism they interact with, these factors can either increase or decrease the level of health and thus complexity and coherence of the individual system. Nothing is absolutely bad or absolutely good for health in Āyurveda:

> Health and disease have the same source; entities, which in suitable state, generate person, cause various disorders in unsuitable state. (Ćaraka Saṃhitā Sūtra Sthāna 25, 29 in Sharma and Dash 2001).

In this view we can identify one of the major differences between Āyurveda and modern Western medicine that exclusively focus on disease, considering it something to be removed or expelled from the organism. By considering health as the dynamic manifestation of life patterns characterized by different levels of coherence, complexity, and integration distributed along a continuum, Āyurveda focuses on the dynamics of health as a ceaseless process of change and adaptation.

The most immediate practical consequence of this view is the relevance attributed to primary prevention that calls into play individual responsibility and awareness. Health is not dependent upon the absence of disease, but it rather derives from everyday life, actions, and behaviors. However, individuals do not live in a vacuum. Health results from the interaction between a complex adaptive system – the individual – and the environmental demands. Therefore, the ecosystem and its balance become substantial determinants of the individual level of health. In addition, considering the social nature of humans and their tendency to develop culture (Baumeister 2005), the notion of environment needs to be broadened to include social relations and cultural artifacts (Massimini and Delle Fave 2000). Overall, prevention is both an individual and collective task, whose outcomes affect persons, communities, and the surrounding nature.

A further implication of the Ayurvedic approach to health concerns the management of chronic conditions. The failure of modern medicine to effectively deal with these situations is mainly due to its prominent focus on the dysfunctions brought about by chronic conditions, rather than on the optimization of the functions and resources available at that level of health. The emphasis on resource empowerment and development has extremely positive consequences on the individual psychophysical well-being, as clearly highlighted in the recent WHO Report on Disability (2011) and in a large amount of studies in the domain of health psychology (see Chap. 9 for an overview). It increases patients' adherence to treatments, motivation and engagement in daily life, quality of interpersonal relations, and social integration. However, these research evidences are not yet integral part of the current health care in the Western medical system.

Overall, health according to Āyurveda is a relative condition, rather than an absolute and discrete state. It is a dynamic process, and at its highest level it is the expression of a highly negentropic pattern of organization emerging from the optimal balance and coherence of a complex living system. Within the Indian view, at the macrocosmic level the universe as a whole is a complex interconnected system of relationships among unmanifest and manifest components of reality; health is the prominent expression of the harmonization and integration among the various components of the individual as a complex interconnected system at the microcosmic level. No contradiction can be detected between this view and the most recent Western conceptualizations of reality outlined in the previous sections. On the contrary, the deep analogies identified between these two views encourage to broaden our culture-bound horizons in the pursuit of a shared understanding of life.

References

Albrecht, G. L., & Devlieger, P. J. (1999). The disability paradox: High quality of life against all odds. *Social Science & Medicine, 48*, 977–988.
Ayers, S. (1997). The application of chaos theory to psychology. *Theory & Psychology, 7*, 373–398.
Baranger, M. (1999). *Chaos, complexity, and entropy – A physics talk for non-physicists*. http://www.necsi.edu/projects/baranger/cce.pdf. Last Accessed on 20 April 2013.
Baumeister, R. F. (2005). *The cultural animal*. New York: Oxford University Press.
Bickenbach, J. E., Chatterji, S., Badley, E. M., & Űstün, T. B. (1999). Models of disablement, universalism and the international classification of impairments, disabilities and handicaps. *Social Science & Medicine, 48*, 1173–1187.
Bishagratna, K. K. L. (Ed.). (1907). *The Suśruta Saṃhitā*. Calcutta: Bishagratna.
Boyd, R., & Richerson, P. J. (1985). *Culture and the evolutionary process*. Chicago: Chicago University Press.
Chalmers, D. J. (1995). Facing up to the problem of consciousness. *Journal of Consciousness Studies, 2*, 200–219.
Churruca, J., Vigil, L., Luna, E., Ruiz-Galiana, J., & Varela, M. (2008). The route to diabetes: Loss of complexity in the glycemic profile from health through the metabolic syndrome to type 2 diabetes. *Diabetes, Metabolic Syndrome and Obesity, 1*, 3–11.
Couture, M. (2007). *Complexity and chaos – State-of-the-art; Overview of theoretical concepts*. Quebec: Defence R&D Canada TM Valcartier.
Dasgupta S. (1922). *A history of Indian philosophy* (5 vol.). Cambridge: Cambridge University Press.
Dasgupta, S. (1924). *Yoga as philosophy and religion*. London: Kegan Paul, Trench, Trubner & Co., Ltd.
Dauwels, J., Srinivasan, K., Ramasubba, R. M., Musha, T., Vialatte, F., Latchoumane, C., Jeong, J., & Cichocki, A. (2011). Slowing and loss of complexity in Alzheimer's EEG: Two sides of the same coin? *International Journal of Alzheimer's Disease*. Article ID 539621, 10 pp doi:*i*
Delle Fave, A. (2006). The impact of subjective experience on the quality of life: A central issue for health professionals. In M. Csikszentmihalyi & I. Csikszentmihalyi (Eds.), *A life worth living: Contributions to positive psychology* (pp. 262–290). New York: Oxford University Press.
Delle Fave, A. (2010). Development through disability: The unfolding and sharing of psychological resources. In G. W. Burns (Ed.), *Happiness, healing and enhancement: Your casebook collection for applying positive psychology in therapy* (pp. 88–99). Hoboken: Wiley.
Delle Fave, A., & Fava, G. A. (2011). Positive psychotherapy and social change. In R. Biswas-Diener (Ed.), *Positive psychology as social change* (pp. 267–292). Dordrecht: Springer Science.
Delle Fave, A., & Massimini, F. (2005). The relevance of subjective wellbeing to social policies: Optimal experience and tailored intervention. In F. Huppert, N. Baylis, & B. Keverne (Eds.), *The science of wellbeing* (pp. 379–404). Oxford: Oxford University Press.
Delle Fave, A., Massimini, F., & Bassi, M. (2011). *Psychological selection and optimal experience across cultures*. Dordrecht: Springer Science.
Duke, M. P. (1994). Chaos theory and psychology: Seven propositions. *Genetic, Social, and General Psychology Monographs, 120*, 265–286.
Eckman, J. P., & Ruelle, D. (1985). Ergodic theory of chaos and strange attractors. *Review of Modern Physics, 57*, 617–656.

Edwards, R., Beuter, A., & Glass, L. (1999). Parkinsonian tremor and simplification in network dynamics. *Bulletin of Mathematical Biology, 51*, 157–177.

Eldredge, N., & Grene, M. (1992). *Interactions: The biological context of social systems.* New York: Columbia University Press.

Engel, G. L. (1977). The need for a new medical model: A challenge for biomedicine. *Science, 196*, 129–136.

Fromm, J. (2004). *The emergence of complexity*. Kassel: Kassel University Press GmbH.

Fromm, J. (2005). *Types and forms of emergence*. Kassel: Kassel University Press GmbH. http://arxiv.org/abs/nlin.AO/0506028

Goldberger, A. L., Amaral, L. A., Hausdorff, J. M., Inanov, P., Peng, C. K., & Stanley, H. E. (2002a). Fractal dynamics in physiology: Alterations with disease and aging. *Proceedings of the National Academy of Science USA, 99*, 2466–2472.

Goldberger, A. L., Peng, C. K., & Lipsitz, A. (2002b). What is physiologic complexity and how does it change with aging and disease? *Neurobiology of Aging, 23*, 23–26.

Goldstein, J. (1999). Emergence as a construct: History and issues. *Emergence, 1*, 49–72.

Hausdorff, J. M., Mitchell, S. L., & Firtion, R. (1997). Altered fractal dynamics of gait. *Journal of Applied Physiology, 82*, 262–269.

Holden, A., & Muhamad, M. (1986). A graphical zoo of strange and peculiar attractors. In A. Holden (Ed.), *Chaos*. Manchester: Manchester University Press.

Holland, J. H. (1995). *Hidden order: How adaptation builds complexity*. Reading: Addison-Wesley.

Holland, J. H. (1997). Emergence. *Philosophica, 59*, 11–40.

Holland, J. H. (1998). *Emergence: From chaos to order*. Oxford: Oxford University Press.

Hood, L., & Flores, M. (2012). A personal view on systems medicine and the emergence of proactive P4 medicine: Predictive, preventive, personalized and participatory. *New Biotechnology, 29*(6), 613–624. doi:10.1016/j.nbt.2012.03.004.

Ingstad, B. (1999). The myth of disability in developing nations. *The Lancet, 354*, 757–758.

Jablonka, E., & Lamb, M. J. (2005). *Evolution in four dimensions. Genetic, epigenetic, behavioural and symbolic variation in the history of life*. Cambridge, MA: MIT Press.

Kaplan, D. T., Furman, M., & Pincus, S. M. (1991). Aging and complexity of cardiovascular dynamics. *Biophysics Journal, 59*, 945–949.

Kaufman, S. (2008). *Reinventing the sacred. A new view of science, reason and religion*. New York: Basic Books.

Keyes, C. L. M. (2007). Promoting and protecting mental health as flourishing: A complementary strategy for improving national mental health. *American Psychologist, 62*, 95–108.

Khalil, E. L., & Boulding, K. E. (Eds.). (1996). *Evolution, order and complexity*. New York: Routledge.

Kresh, J. Y., & Izrailtyan, I. (1998). Evolution in functional complexity of heart rate dynamics. *American Journal of Physiology, 275*, R720–R727.

Kuppuswami, B. (1977). *Dharma and society*. New Delhi: McMillan.

Kyriazis, M. (2003). Practical applications of chaos theory to the modulation of human ageing: Nature prefers chaos to regularity. *Biogerontology, 4*, 75–90.

Mangel, M. (2001). Complex adaptive systems, aging and longevity. *Journal of Theoretical Biology, 213*, 559–571.

Manor, B., & Lipsitz, L. A. (2012). Physiologic complexity and aging: Implications for physical function and rehabilitation. *Progress in Neuro-Psychopharmacology & Biological Psychiatry*, S0278-5846(12)00239-4. doi:10.1016/j.pnpbp.2012.08.020

Manor, B., Costa, M. D., Hu, K., Newton, E., Starobinets, O., Kang, H. G., Peng, C. K., Novak, V., & Lipsitz, L. A. (2010). Physiological complexity and system adaptability: Evidence from postural control dynamics of older adults. *Journal of Applied Physiology, 109*, 1786–1791.

Massimini, F., & Delle Fave A. (2000). Individual development in a bio-cultural perspective. *American Psychologist, 55*, 24–33.

Maturana, H., & Varela, F. (1986). *The tree of knowledge: A new look at the biological roots of human understanding*. Boston: New Science Library.

Mazzocchi, F. (2012). Complexity and the reductionism-holism debate in systems biology. *WIREs Systems Biology and Medicine*. doi:10.1002/wsbm.1181.

Meyers, A. R., Anderson, J. J., Miller, D. R., Shipp, K., & Hoenig, H. (2002). Barriers, facilitators and access for wheelchair users: Substantive and methodologic lessons from a pilot study of environmental effects. *Social Science & Medicine, 55*, 1435–1446.

Miller, J. G. (1970). *Living systems*. New York: McGraw-Hill.

Monod, J. (1971). *Chance and necessity: An essay on the natural philosophy of modern biology*. New York: Knopf.

Morandi, A., Tosto, C., Sartori, G., & Roberti di Sarsina, P. (2010). Advent of a link between Āyurveda and modern health science. In *Proceedings of the First International Congress on Āyurveda, "Āyurveda: The Meaning of Life – Awareness, Environment, and health"*, Milan, Italy, 21–22 Mar 2009. Evidence Based Complementary and Alternative Medicine. 2011:929083. doi:10.1155/2011/929083. Epub 2010 Oct 17

Morandi, A., Tosto, C., Roberti di Sarsina, P., & Dalla Libera, D. (2011). Salutogenesis and Āyurveda: Indications for public health management. *The EPMA Journal, 2*, 459–465.

Nicolis, G., & Prigogine, I. (1989). *Exploring complexity*. New York: Freeman & Co.

Prabhavananda, S. (1977). *Spiritual heritage of India*. Madras: Sri Ramakrishna Math.

Prigogine, I., & Stengers, I. (1984). *Order out of chaos*. New York: Bantam.

Rao, K. R. (2008). Prologue: Introducing Indian psychology. In K. R. Rao, A. C. Paranjpe, & A. K. Dalal (Eds.), *Handbook of Indian psychology* (pp. 1–18). New Delhi: Cambridge University Press India.

Rioux, J. (2012). A complex, nonlinear dynamic systems perspective on Āyurveda and Ayurvedic research. *Journal of Alternative and Complementary Medicine, 18*, 709–718.

Saracci, R. (1997). The World Health Organization needs to reconsider its definition of health. *British Medical Journal, 314*, 1409.

Schierwagen, A. K. (1987). Dendritic branching patterns. In H. Degn & A. V. Holden (Eds.), *Chaos in biological systems*. New York: Plenum Press.

Sharma, R. K., & Dash, B. (Eds.). (2001). *Ćaraka Saṃhitā*. Varanasi: Chaukhamba Sanskrit Series Office.

Simeonsson, R. J., Lollar, D., Hollowell, J., & Adams, M. (2000). Revision of the international classification of impairments, disabilities, and handicaps. Developmental issues. *Journal of Clinical Epidemiology, 53*, 113–124.

Skinner, J. E., Molnar, M., Vybiral, T., & Mitra, M. (1992). Applications of chaos theory to biology and medicine. *Integrative Physiology and Behavioral Science, 27*, 39–53.

Sodergren, S. C., & Hyland, M. E. (2000). What are the positive consequences of illness? *Psychology and Health, 15*, 85–97.

Srikantha Murthy, K. R. (Ed.). (2007a). *Vaghbata Astanga Hrdayam*. Varanasi: Chowkhamba Krishnadas Academy.

Srikantha Murthy, K. R. (Ed.). (2007b). *Suśruta Saṃhitā Sūtra Sthāna*. Varanasi: Chowkhamba Krishnadas Academy.

Thirumulpadu, V. K. R. (2010). *Glimpses of wisdom*. Bangalore: I-AIM.

Tononi, G., & Edelman, G. M. (1998). Consciousness and complexity. *Science, 282*, 1846–1851.

Ünalan, H., Gençosmanoğlu, B., Akgün, K., Karamehmetoğlu, Ş., Tuna, H., Önes, K., Rahimpenah, A., Uzun, E., & Tüzün, F. (2001). Quality of life of primary caregivers of spinal cord injury survivors living in the community: Controlled study with short form-36 questionnaire. *Spinal Cord, 39*, 318–322.

Űstün, T. B., Chatterji, S., Bickenbach, J. E., Trotter, R. T., II, Room, R., Rehm, J., & Saxena, S. (Eds.). (2001). *Disability and culture. Universalism and diversity*. Göttingen: Hogrefe and Huber Publishers.

Valiathan, M. S. (2009). *The Legacy of Ćaraka*. Hyderabad: Universities Press.

Wilson, E. O. (1975). *Sociobiology: The new synthesis*. Harvard: Bellknap.

World Health Organization. (1978). *Declaration of Alma-Ata: International conference on primary health care*, Alma-Ata. http://www.who.int/hpr/NPH/docs/declaration_almaata.pdf

World Health Organization. (2011). *World report on disability 2011*. http://whqlibdoc.who.int/publications/2011/9789240685215_eng.pdf

Conclusions

Chapter 11
Joining Knowledge Traditions: Towards an Integrated Approach to Health and Well-Being

Antonio Morandi, A.N. Narayanan Nambi, and Antonella Delle Fave

This book was conceived as an attempt to bring together Western and Indian approaches to the theme of health care and promotion, with the aim to propose an integrated perspective that can help overcome the limitations of culture-bound models and highlight the contribution potential of a complex and multidimensional view to research and intervention practices.

As described in the first part of this book, during the twentieth century the focus of Western medicine on illness care rather than on health care led to a substantial neglect of prevention practices in favor of an almost exclusive attention to overt physical symptoms and signs that can be objectively measured, exacerbated by the necessity to cope with an increasing shortage of financial resources. Only recently researchers and practitioners started considering the subjective perception of health and the influence of mental conditions on physical functioning as crucial determinants of health that must be scientifically studied and evaluated.

The bio-psycho-social model, developed with the aim of gathering the biological, psychological, and social factors that influence health under a unifying framework, is however still in its infancy. The difficulties in operationalizing it at both the research and intervention levels are mainly derived from the typical fragmentation of knowledge that characterizes Western culture.

A. Morandi (✉)
Ayurvedic Point, Milano, Italy
e-mail: dr.morandi@ayurvedicpoint.it

A.N. Narayanan Nambi
SNA Oushadhasala Pvt. Ltd, Thrissur, Kerala, India
e-mail: drnambi@hotmail.com

A. Delle Fave
Department of Pathophysiology and Transplantation,
University of Milano, Milan, Italy
e-mail: antonella.dellefave@unimi.it

A. Morandi and A.N. Narayanan Nambi (eds.), *An Integrated View of Health and Well-being*, Cross-Cultural Advancements in Positive Psychology 5, DOI 10.1007/978-94-007-6689-1_11,

In order to overcome these difficulties, a conceptual shift is required, from the understanding of health as a utopian goal or an extraordinary condition to be artificially achieved to the expression of a natural condition to be preserved. This approach characterizes most traditional knowledge systems, including Āyurveda, the system of medicine developed in the Indian subcontinent that is taken in this book as an exemplary model. The integration of the two approaches may generate a novel conceptualization of health and health care that could lead to fruitful outcomes at both the research and practice levels.

The possibility of this integration emerges from the recurrence of some common elements recurring across the different chapters, briefly summarized as follows:

1. Health can be conceptualized as a condition of coherence emerging from the network of interrelated functions that characterizes any living being as a complex adaptive system. It accounts for the system's resilience and adaptability to the environmental variations.
2. Increasing levels of global coherence in an organism are related to higher levels of balance, self-sufficiency, resilience, and thus health. However, since organisms are dissipative structures, they need to actively exchange information with the environment in order to maintain their coherence. This information is represented by food at the physical level and by memes – cultural instructions and rules, behavioral and interaction patterns, and outcomes of mental processes (Richerson and Boyd 2005; Massimini and Delle Fave 2000) – at the psychological level. Such a multifaceted information exchange can be broadly described as the transformation of heterologous items into homologous ones through nutrition, breathing, and sense-mediated perception. The global quality of the information exchange with environment thus represents an indicator of the system's health.
3. Health is a dynamic phenomenon rather than the opposite pole of disease. As a process of adaptation to environmental conditions, it undergoes continuous variations. From this perspective disease can be understood as a progressive decrease in the living system's resilience levels that can lead to different balance configurations, progressively more distant from the optimal one but nevertheless compatible with life – as happens in chronic conditions. This conceptualization emphasizes preservation of a healthy balance, rather than intervention against disease, as the key factor of prevention. Accordingly, cure itself should aim at strengthening and possibly increasing residual levels of health and balance, rather than only attack disease. In this model the definition of disease changes as well, from a discrete and alien condition to be fought to an idiopathic condition of suboptimal health.
4. Historical, cultural, social, and economic factors contribute to build the conceptual framework in which health and disease are interpreted. The biomedical view of medicine, based on the health-disease opposition, is grounded into the epistemological methodology of the binary system. The binary system has been characterizing the history of Western thought, language, and worldview (Derrida 1978). It is centered on the clear-cut definition and juxtaposition of two theoretical opposites such as presence/absence, male/female, life/death, and health/disease,

often implying a value hierarchy between the "positive" and the "negative" pole. The binary opposition is built on "discontinuity rather than continuity" (Goody 1977, p. 81). Focusing on discontinuity is indeed beneficial in articulating crystal clear categories, especially within disciplines such as the biomedical ones, where organization and structure are helpful tools to describe the dynamics of living systems. However, it runs the risk of an all-out dichotomization and hierarchical organization of reality (Soosai-Nathan and Delle Fave in press). Although quantum mechanics and systems biology have provided empirical evidence of the limitations of this perspective, it is still dominating in the medical model, and it substantially influences health representations and clinical practice. On the contrary the Indian tradition, within which Āyurveda developed, is grounded into the perspective of interconnectedness, as clearly elucidated throughout the second part of this book.

5. Health represents a natural and basic condition, not a plus. Full health is the optimal expression of each individual living being, and it is variably expressed according to the individual's specific balance and resilience potential. Conditions of lower health may arise, while the health optimal baseline that characterizes each organism cannot be exceeded.
6. Health is the outcome of the individual's active process of interaction and exchange with the environment, and consciousness represents a crucial factor for preserving its balance and optimality. The level of individual awareness substantially influences mind-set, daily behavior, and lifestyle, thus contributing to define the degree of the person's adaptation and resilience. As a matter of fact, the healthy individual in Āyurveda is *Svastha*, the one who is centered into his/her self, a definition encompassing self-awareness and agency. Interestingly, the Indian system emphasizes the primacy of a ground level of self-awareness, related to *ātman*, that underlies the self-awareness level related to individual identity, considered instead the ground level in Western psychology. The *ātman-related* self-awareness allows for the acknowledgement of the individual's substantial interconnection with the nature and with the universe, thus overcoming the self vs. other polarization attitude. In spite of this crucial difference, the importance of the spiritual dimension in well-being promotion is also recognized in Western health psychology, as highlighted in several chapters.
7. The interpretation of health and human functioning proposed by Āyurveda (and by other Eastern traditions) can be fruitfully described through the conceptual framework of complex adaptive systems. The identification of a shared model of understanding allows for envisaging an integration between the Western and the Indian systems of knowledge. This may have useful implications for the management of health and disease, facilitating the cross-fertilization and synergy between the two approaches.
8. The active role of individuals in preserving and promoting their own health becomes particularly evident in habits and lifestyle – comprising nutrition, biorhythms' observance, and physical and mental exercise. These behaviors, considered since millennia core dimensions of health by Āyurveda, are currently acknowledged as central to well-being and prevention in Western biomedicine as well.

At the social level, Āyurveda attributes a central role in health promotion to rituals and collective behaviors that often mark developmental passages and encompass health practices. Also the relationship with the natural environment – that represents a primary source of health, offering the whole range of remedies and medicaments used by traditional medicines – gets strengthened by rituals and ceremonies transmitted across generations, together with the practical knowledge embedded in them (evident in the local systems of medicine). This dimension got lost in modern Western medicine, based on synthetic drugs, but it is undergoing a revitalization trend through thermal and wellness treatments, often taking place in natural environments and fostering the adoption of a daily schedule more tuned with the natural rhythms. However, the social and individual value of traditions and rituals can represent an important source of knowledge and well-being promotion in modern society, especially as concerns those rituals and collective behaviors that encompass hygiene and health practices and that are still part of the folk knowledge in most Western countries.

11.1 Implications for Practice and Applied Research

The implications of this perspective for health conceptualization and management are far-reaching, and they involve both prevention and care systems.

11.1.1 Personalization

Both Āyurveda and the latest acquisition of Western medicine highlight the importance of personalizing prevention and treatment programs. As illustrated in several chapters of this book, the western bio-psycho-social model stresses the centrality of the person as a unique and dynamic blend of biological and cultural components and as an active and mindful agent. From the perspective of Ayurveda, each person is constitutionally characterized by a peculiar balance of the three *doṣa* that requires customized intervention aimed at preserving – and if necessary restoring – that specific balance pattern.

According to both approaches, this individual uniqueness must be reflected in person-tailored intervention programs. There are several conceptual and operational differences however in the way this assumption is translated into practice.

In Āyurveda, the personalization of treatment/prevention practice logically derives from the conceptual framework, typological classification, and diagnostic procedures the medical practice relies upon. Personalization has been structurally characterizing this system of medicine since its foundations. In the Western medicine, personalization is a very recent acquisition, and it is juxtaposed to a whole tradition of standardized, protocol-based, and disease-centered procedures. Therefore, it presently represents a laudable aspiration rather than a common practice, due to the lack of clear-cut conceptual underpinnings and empirically grounded diagnostic and therapeutic tools. Advancements in genetics have provided some insight into individual differences at the biological and physiological levels that can orient pharmacological treatment choices. However, this approach is in its infancy, and its effective development will depend upon investment of large amounts of money, time, and research resources. Moreover, it only focuses on one of the three dimensions of the person, neglecting the psychological and social components.

The Ayurvedic view of the individual is conceptually parsimonious and intrinsically dynamic. The *doṣa* imbalance gets reflected at the various levels of the person's system, and it is possible therefore to treat it by means of few systemic intervention tools, effective at the various levels simultaneously. Moreover, the *doṣa* balance undergoes changes across the different life stages, therefore allowing for an even more fine-tuned intervention that takes into account not only the person's *prakṛti* but also her age and life stage. The Western approach to personalization is instead substantially fragmented into sealed off, separated practices at the various levels of the person's system involving different practitioners who often neither know each other nor the other's discipline and intervention practices. Moreover, in the lack of a unifying and systemic view, interventions are basically still disease focused, even within the domain of personalized pharmacotherapy.

11.1.2 Interconnection

A convergence between the two perspectives in the domain of health management is largely desirable, in view of its potential implications at various levels of intervention:

The body/mind interplay. In spite of the laudable efforts of the psychosomatic approach, the Western medical practice is still based on knowledge fragmentation, and the lack of a unifying model does not allow the general practitioner to take in due account the interplay between mind and body. Āyurveda provides instead a comprehensive approach to such interaction, and some of its concepts and models – such as *Tridoṣa* and *Triguṇa* – can usefully complement the Western approach to diagnosis and care, in order to achieve an authentically psychophysical description of the individual.

The person/environment interplay. Although the bio-psycho-social model acknowledges the influence of environmental factors on health, it substantially focuses on the social dimension and considers it prominently in terms of standard of living, equality/inequality in the access to health care, gender roles, and education. Moreover, the model is grounded into a monocultural, Western perspective that does not consider national and cultural variations in the representations of health and in the social actions undertaken to promote it. Āyurveda provides a more articulated and at the same time exhaustive view of this interplay, distinguishing its occurrence at various levels:

(a) *The bioecological level.* The importance of the natural environment emerges in the concept of *kalapariṇāma* as a major source of disease and in the importance attributed to the use of local foods and medicaments in order to most effectively preserve and restore health. These aspects are largely neglected in the Western lifestyle, though a more careful consideration of them would substantially improve citizens' health and quality of life – for example, through a daily organization more consistent with biorhythms or nutrition habits in harmony with local and seasonal food availability.
(b) *The sociocultural level.* Attention to sociocultural differences is steadily growing in the Western social sciences – such as economics, sociology, and psychology. Much less emphasis is put on these factors in the domain of health care; more specifically, no systematic attempts have been made to comprehensively describe the individual-community interplay as regards health and to provide directions for harmonizing it. By including rituals and relationships in its model of health, Āyurveda offers a pathway towards a clearer evaluation of these factors in health promotion and management.
(c) *The transcendental level.* In the Western view the spiritual dimension is considered a useful tool to promote health, in light of its benefits at the psychological and lifestyle levels. It nevertheless remains a private issue that may or may not be part of the individual's reality, without substantial implications for health management. On the contrary, the Indian vision endorsed by Āyurveda locates the spiritual dimension at the core of individual life: *Ātman* and *ānandamayakosha* are substantive components of any living system and of the universe at the same time. From this perspective, the spiritual dimension is not a matter of personal belief and choice, but it represents the ultimate reality. It therefore occupies a central place in the promotion of health as global balance and fullness. This approach is common to most non-Western traditions. However, its implications for health are rooted into personal adherence and choice, and it is very difficult to envisage their generalizability. Anyway, its role in providing individuals with a worldview characterized by substantial interconnectedness is surely crucial to orient behaviors, meaning-making processes, attitudes towards life and death, health and disease, self, and others.

The culture interplay. As repeatedly stated throughout this book, cultural cross-fertilization can generate a more complex view of health and well-being, allowing to overcome culture boundaries and to expand our understanding of human life and functioning. A vision of reality that encompasses different perspectives in a unitary and global framework can only provide benefits to our knowledge of the processes that underlie the unfolding of life and health, presently threatened by a strong fragmentation tendency. A broader outlook based on the emphasis on commonalities rather than on differences and the identification of models facilitating the integration of knowledge across cultures – such as the complex adaptive system model proposed in this volume – can generate deep awareness of the network of interconnections in which humans are immersed.

References

Derrida, J. (1978). *Writing and difference* (A. Bass, Trans.). London/New York: Routledge.
Goody, J. (1977). *The domestication of the savage mind*. Cambridge: Cambridge University Press.
Massimini, F., & Delle Fave, A. (2000). Individual development in a bio-cultural perspective. *American Psychologist, 55*, 24–33.
Richerson, P. J., & Boyd, R. (2005). *Not by genes alone. How culture transformed human evolution*. Chicago: University of Chicago Press.
Soosai-Nathan, L., & Delle Fave, A. (in press). The altruism spiral: An integrated model for a harmonious future. In H. Marujo & L. M. Neto (Eds.), *Building positive nations and communities*. Dordrecht: Springer.

Index

A. Morandi and A.N. Narayanan Nambi (eds.), *An Integrated View of Health and Well-being*, Cross-Cultural Advancements in Positive Psychology 5, DOI 10.1007/978-94-007-6689-1,

MIX
Papier aus verantwortungsvollen Quellen
Paper from responsible sources
FSC® C105338

If you have any concerns about our products,
you can contact us on
ProductSafety@springernature.com

In case Publisher is established outside the EU,
the EU authorized representative is:
Springer Nature Customer Service Center GmbH
Europaplatz 3, 69115 Heidelberg, Germany

Printed by Libri Plureos GmbH
in Hamburg, Germany